"What an exciting and [...] offers helpful and unique ways to move from being a bystander in life to a full-on participant. ... Blending her own experiences with tried-and-true meditation and mindfulness techniques, she offers us easy and accessible ways to be joyful and present and to find peace and quiet in our lives every day."
— Beryl Bender Birch, director and founder of The Hard & The Soft Yoga Institute and The Give Back Yoga Foundation

"You can tell that Cara Bradley walks her talk. Her advice on mindful movement comes from lived experience, and it's not about having a big special project in addition to everything else you're doing. It's about how to incorporate movement and meditation into the life you already have. Whoever you are — an athlete, a mom who runs a business, a retiree — there's something here for you."
— Barry Boyce, editor in chief of *Mindful* magazine and Mindful.org

"*On the Verge* is a compelling book of wisdom and practicality that supports all of us on this journey of life. In her book, Cara Bradley reveals teachings that empower us to address our roadblocks and embrace life from a real and grounded approach."
— Kelly McNelis, founder of Women for One

"If you've ever longed to tap into the power and energy of your very best moments again and again, Cara Bradley will show you how. *On the Verge* helps you access your natural potential and shine brightly in all aspects of your life."
— Bryant McGill, internationally bestselling author of *Voice of Reason* and United Nations Global Champion

"*On the Verge* is a book about the essence of living fully. In straightforward language packed with supportive examples, Cara Bradley offers practices and strategies that liberate your attention from the consternations of a busy mind so that all your energy, attention, and care are available to inform your ongoing emergence into the future. I have no doubt that those who follow the advice in this book will discover the wonder and joy of a life fully lived."

— Jeff Carreira, author of *The Soul of a New Self: Embracing the Future of Being Human*

"Every coach and athlete knows that it takes more than advice to succeed, and Cara Bradley goes beyond the usual advice giving. She points you to the place within where you already know how to tap your personal power and thrive in every moment of every day."

— Andy Talley, head coach of Villanova University football and AFCA Coach of the Year

"*On the Verge* offers the most practical and useful advice on how to live in the present moment in complete awareness of reality, good or bad, and how best to be with that awareness, rather than resisting it and suffering the consequences of doing so."

— Philip Micali, founder and principal, bWell International, Inc.

"Daily practices designed for well-being, health, and happiness can get us out of our emotional ruts and disrupt our usual habits. But sometimes even these practices slip into the realm of regimen and routine. Why do we not notice? Why don't we pay attention? *Why do we keep falling asleep?* In this book, Cara Bradley gives us much-needed insights on how to keep our practices sharp and our attitude alert. The core question that drives this book is 'How can we be most alive in every single moment?' Cara provides us with Primer Practices and Gut Checks we can use to keep tuning up our daily practice and stepping up our game."

— Bonnitta Roy, founder of Alderlore Insight Center, associate editor of *Integral Review* journal, and Master of Arts in Consciousness Studies program coordinator at the Graduate Institute

ON THE VERGE

ON THE VERGE

Wake Up, Show Up, and Shine

CARA BRADLEY

New World Library
Novato, California

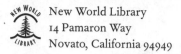 New World Library
14 Pamaron Way
Novato, California 94949

Text design by Tona Pearce Myers

Library of Congress Cataloging-in-Publication Data is available.

First printing, April 2016
ISBN 978-1-60868-375-8
EISBN 978-1-60868-376-5
Printed in Canada on 100% postconsumer-waste recycled paper

 New World Library is proud to be a Gold Certified Environmentally Responsible Publisher. Publisher certification awarded by Green Press Initiative. www.greenpressinitiative.org

10   9   8   7   6   5   4   3   2   1

For Brian, Christina, and Julianna — the bright stars who light my path and help me to show up and shine

Contents

Part III: Verge Practices

Part IV: Verge Strategies

Part V: Show Up and Shine

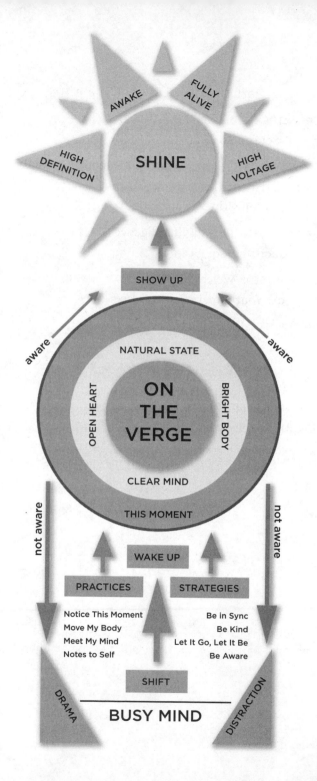

Introduction

I was nineteen years old when I stepped up to the starting line for my last college track race, with no clue that my life would be forever changed. On that auspicious day, I managed to settle down, show up, and — with surprising grace — sail across the finish line in record time. In two minutes and change, I went from ordinary runner to elite athlete. In a flash, I experienced a surge of strength that didn't come from merely trying harder but, instead, seemed to emerge from a place where I felt clear, powerful, and fully alive.

Prior to that race, I rarely took the time to properly prepare for competition and often crawled to the starting line crippled with prerace jitters. Since it was my last race, I felt I owed it to myself to go out on top and to try my hardest to beat my long-standing personal record. And so, on this day of my last college race, I went for a warm-up jog by myself during which I repeated out loud, "Personal best, personal best."

During my track career, my fastest race was mildly respectable, but by no means exceptional. I trained hard, but not superhard. I was competitive, but not that competitive. I was, at best, an average runner. But I knew I had more in me. My strength was there. Somewhere. What I didn't know was how to access and use it.

I stepped up to the starting line that day unusually calm. I focused on the track ahead, waiting for the starting gun. *Bang*. I took off. On my first lap, I felt completely awake — sort of as if the lights in every cell in my body had suddenly turned on. I felt supercharged with energy. On my second lap, my mind cleared, time slowed, and I became conscious of every step and breath. I passed our top mid-distance runner, forgetting that I was supposed to be average.

As I crossed the finish line, my teammates jumped on me. I had no idea why. What just happened? Personal record? What, six seconds off my record? Hold on... What did I just do? My first reaction was "Wow! I did it! A new personal best for me!" But in the very next moment, a surge of *"Are you kidding me?"* took over my entire body.

Although I felt proud of my race, I also felt disappointed that it had taken me my entire track career to find my inner strength and break my long-standing record. When the rush of excitement settled, the big questions began to mount.

Why had I doubted my ability for so many years? Why hadn't I ever felt that strong in prior races? Where did that incredible charge of energy and sense of aliveness come from? And, most important, *how do I find it again?*

Deep down I felt certain that breaking my personal record was related to my prerace jog. Repeating "Personal best" had settled me. I'd shifted into a relaxed yet alert state where I had no doubt and no fear. In this state, beyond thinking, I soared and I shined. Immediately, I wanted to understand what exactly I'd done to feel that awake and alive. I had to find a system or discipline to help me feel that clear and confident — all the time. I knew one thing for certain: I wanted more.

After my extraordinary experience on the track, I knew my life would never be the same. During that race, I encountered who I was capable of becoming, and I refused to settle for less by falling back asleep. I became hungry for answers, sparking a lifelong curiosity about my own potential and human potential in general.

Years later my husband, Brian, spent a few weeks in the Amazon jungle working with an indigenous community, during which he explored rivers and tributaries in the most vibrant ecosystem on earth. He traveled throughout its vast river system, often stopping at specific places where two rivers merged into one. These places are revered in the river basin as sacred, because it is at these junctures that plants and wildlife thrive more than in any other area on the river. This special place is called "the verge."

As a human-potential junkie, I was ecstatic to learn that a place like the verge actually existed. Imagine the feeling of living on a verge in the Amazon. It made me wonder if, like the plants and wildlife, the people who live on the verge thrive there too. It made me wonder if there was a verge closer to home, and if such a place or state existed, how I could get there and live there.

I started experimenting with techniques and practices that could help me thrive as if I were living on the verge. I took thousands of yoga classes, sat in meditation for hundreds of hours, spent days in silence, chanted, prayed in sweat lodges, had my chakras cleared, read countless self-help and spiritual books, studied the great world religions, bungee-jumped, zip-lined, and walked on hot coals. I searched for a place like the verge where I could feel as awake and fully alive as I did when I was nineteen.

Intrigued ever since, I've discovered you don't have to go deep into the rain forest to find the verge. It is, in fact, available to you in every moment. It's at your fingertips all the time, because *this moment is the verge.*

In this exact moment there's a gap, a split second of time, when you're not quite in the past and not quite in the future. In this moment you are on a threshold, you are on the verge. Do you feel it?

If you're distracted or busy, you'll miss it. You may speed right by it. *Poof!* Just like that, this gap in time will be gone forever. The verge, by nature, is fleeting and elusive. You can't hold on to it, and you can't search for it. You simply need to show up on the verge — on the threshold between a moment ago and a moment from now.

The verge, this very moment, is not just where your mind and body go through the motions of life; it's also where you feel awake and fully alive.

The verge is not only where nature thrives; it's also where *you* thrive.

The verge is where you wake up, show up, and shine.

On the Verge is based on my own direct experience of being awake and fully alive and on my curiosity about human potential and what it means to thrive. Although I stand on the shoulders of many teachers, the insights I share with you flow from my own investigation and discoveries. My intent for this book was not to try to rehash the words of great masters of philosophy, science, and religion. So you won't find quotations of great sages or references to scientific studies.

I am offering a raw and unfiltered expression of what I have experienced in my own practices and in teaching thousands of people. I attempt to express as simply as possible how it feels to break free of the confines of my own cluttered, often chaotic mind and be conscious in a human body in a busy world. I humbly offer you my experience of what it feels like to wake up, show up, and shine.

On the Verge emerged from my thirty-five years of teaching fitness and yoga and my lifelong dedication to coaching thousands of people to experience life fully — and to do so over and over again. By taking this journey with me, I hope you'll learn to do the same — to adopt a few practices and strategies that will help you show up in this moment and embrace life fully.

On the Verge isn't about changing your body, love life, or finances. In the pages ahead, I'm not going to tell you what to eat, how to exercise, or how to pray. I won't ask you to sit still for hours at a time, nor will I tell you what you need to improve. There's enough advice out there and, in my opinion, the more you read about what you should be doing, the less likely you are to actually commit to anything.

Living on the verge is not about doing more, but about *being* more. It isn't about achieving more; it's about *experiencing* more. It's not about being someone different, as there's no "better version of you" on the horizon. Everything you're searching for is available to you in this moment. Everything you need is right here on the verge.

You'll discover that when you show up in this moment — when you are 100 percent engaged right here and right now — you arrive in a space where you are fully aware. In this space, beyond your busy mind, you glimpse your naturally occurring state of being awake and fully alive. In your natural state your mind is clear, your body bright, and your heart open. On the verge, in your natural state, you show up and shine.

In the pages ahead you'll learn practices and strategies to help you shift your perspective beyond your busy mind, glimpse your natural state, and live on the verge. But don't assume you'll wake up and show up just by reading this book. Don't just hope that somehow you'll be ready to shine when you need to shine most — during the big board meeting or the last play of the game. That kind of thinking is risky business. Don't *hope* you'll miraculously feel awake and fully alive when you want to or need to most. Instead, commit to taking this journey with me and discover through practice what it feels like to show up and live on the verge over and over again.

You are already awake and fully alive. You are already on the verge. You just may not believe it — yet. I want to help you believe in your extraordinary human potential to show up and shine in even the most ordinary moments of your everyday life. I want to help you show up and shine as I did on the track thirty years ago, and to do so not by accident or once in a while, but *on purpose* and all the time. So buckle your seat belts and get ready to break your own records and achieve your own personal best. Let's get started.

PART I

WAKE UP
AND SHOW UP

CHAPTER ONE

"Let Me Do"

I was born Carolyn Marie Ferrara, the only daughter sandwiched between two sons in an Italian American family from the Coney Island section of Brooklyn. As a fiercely independent child, I didn't take orders well, resisted advice, and insisted on doing everything myself. My three favorite words were "Let me do." No one could tell me what to do or show me how to do it. I needed to *do* it myself, thank you very much. My need for autonomy carried through my teenage years, when day in and day out I insisted on being left alone to figure things out for myself.

This "Let me do" attitude worked both for me and against me. I developed some useful skills, such as not believing everything I read, standing up to peer pressure, and possessing a readiness to try most things at least once (as long as it doesn't involve jumping out of planes).

In early adulthood I became impatient and impulsive, making hasty decisions without consulting the experts, a.k.a. my parents, including a last-minute transfer in my sophomore year of college, quitting a sweet position at a New York investment bank, and dropping out of a fast-track MBA program at New York University. I married in my twenties, changed my name to Cara in my thirties, and got a tattoo in my forties. I've taught everything from step aerobics to hip-hop dance, performed on Rollerblades around the world, and started a handful of businesses, including selling hair bows in Greenwich Village, ice-cream cones in New Hampshire, and figure-skating apparel in Nova Scotia.

So here I am, Cara, the "Let me do" risk taker, who must see, hear, taste, smell, and touch everything before I accept it as the real deal. I don't like gimmicks and steer clear of big promises. Don't try to BS me, because I'll smell it a mile away. Before I buy, I need to touch. Before I sell, I need to trust.

Being a "Let me do" kind of girl means I need to experience everything *myself*. When I hug my daughters, I want to *feel* the hug. When I'm chopping garlic for fresh tomato sauce, I want to *smell* the garlic.

The reason I have to thoroughly see, hear, taste, smell, and touch everything is quite simple. When I'm fully engaged in whatever I'm doing, I feel more awake. When I *directly experience* what is happening, I feel fully alive — and, by the way, so do you.

Life Is Not a Spectator Sport

You experience life in different ways. Some experiences are direct, some are secondhand, and some are muted. A *direct experience* is your firsthand knowledge of a sensation, state, or feeling; it's exactly what you're feeling in any given moment through your five senses. *Secondhand experiences* are someone else's interpretation of an event or experience. A *muted experience* occurs when you're mentally distracted or emotionally drained; your experience of life is muddled because it's mediated by your busy mind.

Let's take a closer look at how you may be experiencing life.

Secondhand Experience

A secondhand experience is a description of a sensation, state, or feeling as told, written, or demonstrated by others. It's their interpretation of what's happening. Your mother tells you about the sunset she watched or your friend says the burgers at Sally's Diner are the best she's ever eaten.

Take eating an orange. If your friend Bob tells you about the orange he ate, it's not your firsthand experience — it's secondhand. In other words, Bob's explanation describes his firsthand experience; it won't help you taste the orange.

When I tell people about how invigorated *I feel* after a yoga class, they often smile and nod their heads. They can listen to me all day long, but they'll never, ever know what it's like to practice yoga until they step onto a mat and try it for themselves. My experience won't take them there — ever. It will always be secondhand, that is, until they show up for class.

To use another example. Let's say your friend gives you courtside seats to a basketball game. Sitting on the edge of the action, you hear the players breathing heavily. You feel the wind brush your face as they speed by. However, as close as you are to the game, you're not in the game, and you're not a part of the team. Unless you put on a jersey and step onto the court, you are a spectator experiencing the game secondhand.

Muted Experience

Experiences become muted when you're mentally distracted or emotionally drained. You can say your senses feel fuzzy or foggy. Muted experiences are your muddled interpretation of life through the lens of your busy mind.

For example, you don't notice the sky is blue, because you're consumed with worry about your son's test; you walk past a bunch of roses but their aroma doesn't register, because you're too busy remembering when your ex-husband gave you roses on your anniversary; or you eat an apple but totally miss its crisp tartness, because you're thinking about tomorrow's doctor's appointment.

Most people walk through life having one muted experience after another simply because they're too busy thinking. When you are consumed with overthinking and overdoing, life becomes a string of muted experiences, and over time you grow dull to your five senses. Over time, you grow dull to your natural capacity to directly experience life fully.

Direct Experience

There are moments in life when your experience is direct and vivid. What you see is sharper and clearer, what you touch is more real, tastes are more vibrant, smells are stronger, and sounds are more distinct. These are your direct sensory experiences.

Direct, or firsthand, experiences are moments of deep connection, when you're vividly aware of your sensations, states, and feelings. You experience life beyond the filter of your busy mind in a space where you feel awake and alert. Experience life through the crystal-clear lens of your own direct experience, and your world becomes bright, your senses light up, and you feel fully alive. When you directly experience the moment, you are on the verge.

When you directly experience the moment, you are on the verge.

A direct experience is not something you learn from a book or a teacher. It's your own encounter with reality — with life as it is happening at this very moment. A direct experience is yours and no one else's.

Firsthand, direct experiences happen in present time; they're your full sensory experience of whatever's happening right now. For example, you smell the ocean, you feel cold, or you see the blue sky. Your direct experiences offer you a real-time encounter with life in this exact moment and in high definition.

Direct experiences come in many packages and arrive at the most ordinary moments, like the smell of dinner cooking or the feel of sand between your toes. They can also take your breath away, like hearing your baby say "Mama" for the first time or watching the sun set over the ocean.

You can have a direct experience in any moment. They are happening 24/7. As long as you're breathing, you can tune in to your direct experience of life as it's happening right now.

The only thing holding you back from showing up and directly experiencing your life right now is your busy mind. You're likely conditioned to *do* instead of *feel*, and *think* instead of *be*. Pausing to notice what your five senses are saying may happen more rarely than you'd like to admit. Don't worry, you're not alone. Experiencing life through the muted and sometimes distorted lens of the busy mind is one of our current human dilemmas, one on which I hope to shed some light for you.

The good news is that when you settle down and get out of your own way, your attention drops down below your head and into your body. You'll arrive in a space where you become vividly aware of your senses and exactly what you're seeing, tasting, touching, hearing, and smelling. Connecting with your body through physical sensation is essential to experiencing life fully. Your body *always* experiences life directly and vividly.

This bears repeating. Your body always experiences life directly and vividly. It cannot do otherwise. You can't smell or see something secondhand. Your body is always present; the feeling of grass under your feet cannot be muted or dulled. Only your busy mind can mute or dull your experience.

Since most of us are more identified with what's happening in our minds than in our bodies, we experience most of our lives through the filter of thoughts and emotions. Although your mind is often busy and distracted, your body is always present. In order to directly experience life more often, you'll need

Your body always experiences life directly and vividly.

to shift beyond your busy mind and connect with your body more often. I fully trust you have the potential to do so, and not just once, but all the time.

Pause right now and check in with what's happening. Notice the sensations in your body. What are you feeling, tasting, touching, hearing, and seeing? Take a moment to pause and shift from doing to feeling, from thinking to being. Notice your senses. Show up and engage with life directly, and you'll experience what I call *high-definition, high-voltage living*.

Primer Practices

On the next page is your first Primer Practice. You'll discover many throughout this book. Each only takes a few minutes to do. These easy-to-do Primer Practices will "prime the pump" — they will prep your mind by settling your thoughts and calming your nervous system. As you steady your mind, you shift beyond it into a clear space where you become aware of your body and directly experience your physical sensations.

The Primer Practices are essential to living on the verge. So when you come upon one of them, do yourself a favor and give it a try. I know how easy it is to skip over stuff. The only way you'll truly benefit from what I'm sharing is to roll up your sleeves and get curious about how you're experiencing life. Reading this book may inspire you here and there, but ultimately my words will not help you feel any more awake or any more alive. The Primer Practices are opportunities to do so. Don't just breeze by them.

All of the Primer Practices are available in audio form on the Verge Mobile App, easily downloaded through my website: www.carabradley.net.

Let's do this.

PRIMER PRACTICE:
STOP, TAKE FIVE, EXPERIENCE

This simple exercise couldn't be easier. It's a great way to quickly notice where you are and what you're doing. Practicing this throughout the day can help you become familiar with which experiences of yours are direct, secondhand, or muted. Read the full instructions before starting.

1. Set your timer for two minutes. Close your eyes.
2. Actively pay attention to your breathing, by counting five full breaths. It helps to think, "Inhale, exhale one. Inhale, exhale two, " and so on. Listening to the sound of your breath will almost immediately relax you and begin to settle your busy mind.
3. After five breaths, open your eyes and sit quietly.
4. Try not to put words to your experience. Look around and actively notice your surroundings. What do you see, smell, hear, taste, or touch? If you hear a bird chirp, just note that. Do you smell coffee? Note that too. If your mind is very busy thinking, that's okay too. Whatever you notice is perfect. There are actually no correct answers when you practice — you just practice! Pausing to notice the moment and what you're experiencing is the first step to connecting with your body and waking up to your direct experience more often.

Throughout the day, practice actively paying attention. *Stop, take five, experience.* You can do it in the chaos of your commute, in a moment in between meetings, or while waiting for the school bus to arrive. It is easier to pause when you minimize distractions, but it's not essential. The following situations can help you tune in to your body and notice your direct experience:

Turning off the car radio
Focusing only on finishing the email
Exercising without listening to music
Cooking dinner without trying to multitask

The fact is, if you are breathing, you are experiencing your life. Whether you're aware of what you're experiencing is another matter. I want to help you to become aware of and recognize your direct experiences. Start actively paying attention to what you're experiencing right away. Try it again, right now. Try it several times today. What's happening in this exact moment? What do you see, smell, or hear? How do you feel? Are you tired or energized? Do you feel dull or awake? Start naming your experiences throughout your day.

Naming what you're experiencing gives you breathing space. Pausing to acknowledge sensations interrupts your busy mind and allows you to rest for a moment. Such pauses in the frenzied speed of our everyday lives can be a great relief — like a breath of fresh air.

They also make you available to experience brief moments of beauty or intensity that you've been too distracted to notice. For instance, you may stop at a red light and glance up to notice the sun peeking through the clouds, or you look up from the kitchen sink and catch your daughter dancing by herself in the backyard. Perhaps you take that first bite of a juicy peach and close your eyes to savor its sweetness. I view these brief moments as glimpses of being fully alive.

Such glimpses are happening all the time, and with practice you'll start noticing them in every corner of your life. Glimpses are not just feel-good moments. They are like arriving on the threshold between a moment ago and a moment from now. They are your direct experience in this exact moment.

Glimpses invite you to experience how you're always awake and fully alive. Like a whisper in your ear, they remind you that you already have everything you need to experience your life fully and that you already know how to show up and shine.

Your life is too precious to treat it like a spectator sport, so don't be content to sit courtside watching the game happen in front of you. Why not directly experience your life fully? Let's explore high-definition, high-voltage living. Let's directly experience living on the verge.

Are you ready? I hope so.

Come on, say it out loud with me: *"Let me do!"*

> Glimpses invite you to experience how you're always awake and fully alive.

CHAPTER TWO

On the Verge

As a competitive figure skater, I spent hours on a clean patch of ice practicing figure eights. I traced my figures over and over while on one edge of a very thin blade. I recall drinking in the cold damp air on those early mornings before school in the hushed stillness of the quiet rink. I loved every minute of those training sessions, including the precision of the movement, the serenity of silence, and the joy of being alive.

As a young skater, I became keenly aware of the accuracy required to glide on the edge of a sharp blade. A slight shift in focus or a moment of hesitation would throw my body off just enough to affect the crispness of my edge on the ice. Even a subtle distraction while creating a figure eight could result in the difference between a gold medal and eighth place. There was no room for error. I needed to be *fiercely focused* as I leaned into the edge of my blade. I needed to be fully engaged. Without knowing it then, I was training my mind to recognize when I was distracted and to show up in the moment again and again. I was training to live on the verge.

This Moment Is the Verge

If you're like most people, your mind is busy, filled with untamed emotions and unruly thoughts. Your attention is often anywhere but right here. You churn out thought after thought as you live in the chaos and clutter of your busy mind.

Busy mind is a catchall term I use to include anything that pulls you away from showing up right here and now. Your busy mind includes the thoughts, emotions, stories, and perceptions that often mute your experience and trap you into stressing and overthinking your way through life. Too much mental content frays your nerves and keeps you awake at night. Simply put, your busy mind is an overwhelming place to live. The mental junk drains you; the drama and distraction always leave you feeling exhausted.

Busy mind is a catchall term I use to include anything that pulls you away from showing up right here and now.

Although thinking is useful, overthinking can be detrimental and even destructive. It increases stress and blocks your capacity to connect with your body and access your natural intelligence. But please don't fret. Knowing you have a busy mind is the first step. Get to know your busy mind, and you'll see how too much thinking mutes your experiences.

When you're preoccupied by thoughts and emotions, you experience life through the filtered lens of your busy mind. You see life through the haze of emotional disturbance or the tension of mental stress. If you are living from your busy mind, you're not aware of your body, and if you're not aware of your body, then you're missing the full, direct sensory experience of this very moment — forever.

You are not your busy mind. You are not your thoughts and emotions. When you are settled and stable, you shift beyond your busy mind and directly experience a natural sense of clarity, vitality, and confidence. Beyond your busy mind, you arrive in a space that feels open and vast. You meet life head-on. In this space there are no veils to hide behind and no filters to alter your perspective.

Beyond your busy mind, you experience your natural way of being, a state you'll come to know as clear mind, bright body, and open heart. Beyond your busy mind, you arrive on the verge — where you naturally wake up, show up, and shine.

Verge Yoga

A year after my husband returned home from the Amazon, I opened a yoga center in suburban Philadelphia that I appropriately named Verge Yoga. It was born from my insatiable enthusiasm to experience my life fully. I wanted to share my discoveries with as many people as possible by offering them practices and strategies that would enable them to have their own experiences of being awake and fully alive.

Beyond your busy mind, you experience your natural way of being, a state you'll come to know as clear mind, bright body, and open heart.

Verge Yoga's tagline, "Unblock, Unfold, Unleash," is an ongoing invitation to do just that, to directly experience being awake and fully alive by shifting beyond your busy mind and showing up in the moment — not just once, but all of the time. For the past twelve years, I've been developing a method of synchronizing the mind and body through movement, silence, and stillness that enables students to glimpse their natural state. By slowing down and breathing deeply, students experience high-definition, high-voltage living: they experience themselves beyond their busy mind where they feel clear, energized, and fully alive.

After thousands of hours of my own investigation and just as many hours teaching, I'm ready to offer you my practices and strategies to synchronize your mind and body so that you can have your own empowering direct experiences. I want to help you live on the verge, not once in a while, but every day. Take a look.

Verge Practices: Glimpsing Your Natural State

The Verge Practices are easy-to-use tools to help you get to know your busy mind and shift into the space beyond it, where you glimpse your natural state. During practice, you'll recognize glimpses, short moments, of your natural state of clarity, vitality, and confidence. The practices include:

- *Notice This Moment:* A toolbox of mindfulness exercises to help you recognize your direct experiences in practice and in your daily life; the Primer Practices are all included in this toolbox.
- *Move My Body:* A way to synchronize your mind and body through movement and discover how rhythmic movement settles and calms your mind and nervous system.
- *Meet My Mind:* A way to synchronize your mind and body through silence and stillness and become familiar with how your mind operates.
- *Notes to Self:* Reminders, questions, and intentions to help you consistently wake up, show up, and shine.

Verge Strategies: Living from Your Natural State

The Verge Strategies are more than practices; they help you live in your natural state by staying awake and aware when you would otherwise be stuck in your busy mind, drained by drama, and limited by distraction. These strategies help you navigate your life and maintain balance and energy. The Verge Strategies include:

- *Be in Sync:* Tuning in to your mind and body to maintain clarity and balance, and turning to silence, stillness, and rhythm to stabilize and synchronize.
- *Be Kind:* Making friends with yourself by invoking kindness, tenderness, and humor in your life.
- *Let It Go, Let It Be:* Letting go of your need to force, fix,

or flee in order to become available to experience exactly what is happening in this moment.

- *Be Aware:* Checking in with your mind to notice when you are not aware and to recognize when you are fully aware.

Active versus Passive Attention

As you'll see, the practices and strategies are very helpful in getting to know your busy mind and glimpsing the space beyond it. You're going to practice looking at your busy mind and shifting beyond it over and over. I want to tell you that you don't need practices and strategies to directly experience your life fully. You already have direct experiences all of the time. The catch is that you're just not aware you're having them. To be aware of how you experience this moment, you need to actively pay attention to this moment. In order to show up and directly experience your life, it's important to understand the difference between active attention and passive attention.

In active attention, you're fully right here and right now, with your complete mind and body. Active attention means you notice the dog at the side of the road poised to jump in front of your car; you walk down city streets observing the sights, smells, and sounds; you feel your senses light up with each new experience; and you are fully aware of what you're saying and doing.

In passive attention, you're sort of right here, but sort of distracted or caught up in thoughts that make you feel foggy or dull. You're distracted by the grocery list or plans for dinner, and you don't notice the dog ready to jump. You walk the same streets thinking about this and that, oblivious to the bustle of humanity and the beauty around you.

With active attention, you're aware. With passive attention, you're not aware. When you're aware, you feel alert and engaged in precisely what's happening; you're actively and directly experiencing this moment. When you're not aware, you feel kind of here, sort of present, but also sort of distracted. You may even feel dull. You may notice what's happening around you, but you're not that engaged or curious. Most people shift in and out of being aware, active and passive, all day long. It's important to start noticing if you're active or passive. Let's experience this right now.

 PRIMER PRACTICE:
WAKE-UP CALL

What does it feel like to be here now? This Primer Practice will give you an opportunity to experience the difference between being active and right here and now or passive and sort of here. You can also join me for the guided practice on the Verge Mobile App.

1. Set your timer for two minutes and take a seat.
2. Place your hands on your knees and pause.
3. Don't do anything different. Just sit still and breathe.
4. After two or three breaths, begin to notice what is happening both inside of you and around you.
5. Tune in to your senses. Everything counts in this practice, including noise, physical sensations, smells, the way your clothes feel on your skin, visual stimuli, and even your breath and thoughts.
6. There's no right or wrong. Simply remain curious about what you are experiencing.
7. When your timer goes off, just rest for another few breaths without focusing on anything particular.

Are you active or passive, clear or busy, aware or not aware? Continue to ask yourself this question over and over. Notice when you're more active and aware. Notice when your attention fades and you become passive. Every moment is an invitation to wake up and feel fully alive. Every moment, seemingly big or small, is an opportunity to live on the verge.

You know those big vivid moments, when your world instantly turns upside down, demanding your full attention, and later you seem to remember every sensation. There are pivotal moments, like when a child is born or a loved one passes away; unexpected moments, like when your basement is flooded or you slip on ice; and thrilling moments, like when you receive an unexpected raise, a marriage proposal, or a call that you won the sweepstakes. These moments grab your attention and wake you up — even if you don't want to. But there's more to life than big moments like these. There's a whole game in between them that still needs to be played. It's the moments *in between* that have been the focus of my teaching.

Every day you have opportunities to be awake and actively aware. In fact, every moment is an invitation to directly experience your life fully. Living on the verge is like waking up from a long night's sleep, over and over again, one moment after the next. You actively show up to directly experience life right now, and now, and now. Your senses light up, and you feel awake and fully alive.

CHAPTER THREE

Being Fully Alive

Over the years, I've moved thousands of people through a mix of trendy workouts and ancient practices — and each of them arrived with expectations of getting fit, losing weight, building six-pack abs, and finding peace. I've always sensed, however, that there's a deeper reason for all the striving and searching than just having a great body and a stress-free life. I've sensed that at the root of the search is our innate desire to feel fully alive.

We go to great lengths and great expense to feel fully alive. We'll jump from fad to fad searching for the next best way to feel more empowered or energized. We open our hearts and wallets to what the hippest experts recommend and what the hottest celebrities are doing — all to feel fully alive. I know this because I've been on the same path, searching for ways to feel better, look better, and be better, when underneath all the forcing and fixing I've really just longed to feel more alive.

After a few decades with no earth-shattering results, I called off the search. I let go of needing to feel any different or look any better and gave myself permission to live my life, raise my daughters, teach yoga, and enjoy my husband and friends. It was an incredible relief. My shift in perspective — from seeking to allowing, from doing to being — enabled me to experience space in my life beyond busyness and drama, a space where I experienced

an incredible sense of freedom. It felt like falling back on my bed
and resting my head on my pillow after a long, busy day.

I began to pay attention to my direct experiences, and more
and more I began to glimpse a more natural and authentic way
of living. Shifting my perspective from searching to simply living allowed me to get crystal clear about what was necessary to
fully participate in my life — and not to waste one more second
doing anything less. The trees looked greener, food tasted better,
I felt happier. In this space, beyond the search outside myself, I
unleashed a new sense of joy that touched every area of my life.
Letting go of the need to figure out my life liberated me not only
to show up and experience my life, but to feel fully alive. Beyond
the search, I became familiar with how to live my life in high definition and with high-voltage energy.

Seeing Your World in High Definition

Right here, in this moment, you have the opportunity to fully engage in what's happening, to participate in reading these words,
to feel the couch beneath you or the sun on your face. Show up
right now beyond busyness and actively pay attention, and you
directly experience more of, well, everything. You
feel awake to what's happening around you and
alive to what's happening inside you. Beyond
your busy mind you experience life in high
definition.

High-definition living
is a way to engage
in the world
with all your senses.

High-definition living is a way to engage
in the world with all your senses. It feels crisp
and clear. It's like seeing life as if you were a child
again, when you stared at clouds in the sky and devoured books and movies (along with cookies and candy) with
gusto. Directly experience life in high definition, and you recognize the smallest details of life — the touch of wind tickling

your neck and the smell of wood burning from the fireplace next door.

Now, decades after my final college race, I still vividly remember the details. I clearly remember calmly standing on the starting line waiting for the gun to go off, the smell of spring in the air, and how my spikes felt on the track. I remember everything about that moment — the high-definition experience that redirected my life.

You have your own high-definition moments. Can you think of a few? Perhaps it was the intense emotional high when you got married or the profound disappointment when you didn't get the job. Sometimes these moments are easy to identify, and sometimes they're not as clearly defined. Strengthen your ability to recognize direct experience in the ordinary moments of daily life, and they all go into high definition. The practices you're learning will help you do so — to refine and expand your ability to recognize such high-definition, high-voltage experiences all of the time.

Trying to explain what it means to directly experience life in high definition is like trying to explain how it feels to swim in a cold lake or sing in front of a crowd. It goes beyond words and explanations. As you become more aware of these experiences, you'll ultimately recognize high-definition moments from more of a visceral place, in your body and beyond words. This is important. Remember, your body always experiences the moment directly. Your body senses life firsthand beyond your beliefs, judgments, and conditioning. Your body reveals what's real and true. This is why direct experiences feel precise and complete, and why they often emerge with a resounding "aha."

Snapshots

Because descriptions, even extended ones, cannot capture your whole experience, I'll offer Snapshots, groups of individual words that can serve as instantaneous reminders of the direct experiences in your life. Not every word is going to work for you. My aim is that at least one or two will connect with you. Read these words slowly. Find the ones that resonate. Let them sink in. Draw from these Snapshots in your daily life. They provide you with words to help you recognize your direct experiences.

◉ SNAPSHOT:
A HIGH-DEFINITION EXPERIENCE

Clear	Brilliant	Alive
Bright	Sharp	Ready
Awake	Open	Aware
Alert	Light	Vibrant

Experiencing Life with High-Voltage Energy

There's a powerful energy running through you right now. You can sense it when you're resting or when you're moving. Sometimes you may not feel it at all. When you're engaged in what you're doing, you experience it. When you're hiking, painting, reading, or writing, you feel it. It feels like having the wind at your back and a little extra spring in your step. This high-voltage energy is your aliveness.

High-voltage energy guides you to move and speak. It directs you to slow down and pay attention or encourages you to lean into your boundaries and seek new horizons. Either way, this energy pushes you gently, and sometimes not so gently, to wake up, show up, and participate in life right here and right now.

You've had moments of high-voltage energy; you may simply not have recognized them at the time. Here are a few examples of what high-voltage energy feels like for me:

Seeing the brilliance of the sun as it hits the top of the
    trees in the late afternoon
Hearing the giggles of my neighbor's kids in the backyard
Tasting the crispness of a green apple
Listening deeply to my friend recount a recent crisis
Belting out a song during my commute home
Flying down the hill on my bike

Here's a Snapshot offering you a variety of ways that you
may experience high-voltage energy.

◉ SNAPSHOT:
HIGH-VOLTAGE ENERGY

Excited	Powerful	Charged
Determined	Available	Enthusiastic
Strong	Connected	Fearless
Confident	Curious	

Brand-new students walk through the doors of Verge Yoga
every day, often with a hint of apprehension as they step onto a
yoga mat for the first time. As class begins, they try to breathe
deeply and move slowly. The sweat starts to flow, their bodies
relax, and their minds settle. At the end of class, they take the final
pose, *savasana*, a sweet five-minute rest.

This final pause, in stillness, allows students to let go and
relax. In this space many students experience sensations they
haven't felt in years. It often brings them to tears. They feel their
body come alive, buzzing and tingling from head to toe. They
directly experience a profound sense of ease and peace.

This experience is not random. These students are meeting themselves beyond distraction and drama, and the next time

they practice, they will likely experience it again. You can experience this too, and you never need to step onto a yoga mat to do so.

Mount Cardigan

There's no mistaking high-definition, high-voltage living; experiencing it often stops me in my tracks and makes me pay attention. One such full-sensory encounter happened years ago when I hiked up Mount Cardigan in New Hampshire with friends. Unbeknownst to me, we took the "most challenging" route. Lagging behind the group, I found myself face-to-face with a steep wall of rock, on a cliff no less. Attempting this climb without gear was above my level of expertise, but being the knucklehead that I am, I decided to go for it anyway. As I placed my hands and feet on the sheer rock, my body visibly shook. Step-by-step I climbed, never daring to look down. Although the climb didn't take long, it felt as though it lasted forever.

Finally, I made it to the top and dropped to my knees, dramatically tossing my backpack out of the way. My friends, who had obviously been there a while, casually glanced at me and smiled. It was clear they had no idea what I'd just endured (and I wasn't about to tell them either!). Still shaking and panting, I stretched out on my back and tried to recover.

As I settled down, I noticed a pulsing, a sort of tingling in my arms and legs that spread to my spine and shoulders, then to my head. I felt this wave of energy pulsating from my feet to my face! I felt the sun on my skin, heard the whistle of the wind. I smelled the sweet scent of early spring floating in the air. My body was a symphony of sensations buzzing at high voltage. My senses had lit up, in high definition. I felt fully alive.

When Do You Feel Fully Alive?

High-definition, high-voltage living is right here in this moment, and in this moment, and now in this moment. It's a matter of recognizing when you feel alive. I don't know what makes you feel alive, but you do.

What makes your skin tingle, your heart sing? What makes your mind focus like a laser beam on a target? What transports you beyond your thoughts, drama, and distractions? What makes you feel clear and bright? Is it music, nature, sports? Work? Being with your kids? When do you experience high-voltage energy? What makes you feel fully alive?

I don't know what makes you feel alive, but you do.

I posed these questions to my Facebook friends when asking for help with this chapter. I received dozens of answers, wonderful slices of the everyday human experience. Here are a few responses:

Walking to take in the sun and nature's beauty
When I just *have* to sing
Hiking with my dog
Telling the truth
Knowing my kids are happy
Connecting with people of other cultures and religions
Pushing the final minutes of my run
Sunrises
Giving a compliment to someone I don't know
Feeling the wind
Hearing children's laughter
Feeling in love
Giggling...crying...touching
Laughing until I cry from laughing so hard

As I read through these comments, the words "ordinary" and "available" came to mind. These were everyday experiences. It was remarkable how many comments included water, beaches, nature, and children. None, and I mean not one, of these comments included having more stuff, more money, or six-pack abs. Best of all, these moments of being fully alive were *all* free of charge and commonly available to most of us every day.

Gut Checks

Welcome to your first Gut Check. Gut Checks are inquiries to help you notice what you're doing and how you're living. Found throughout this book, they help you investigate and identify where you're open and available and where you're still stuck in your stories and beliefs. When you come upon a Gut Check, please *just do it*. The only way you'll truly benefit from what I'm sharing is to roll up your sleeves and get curious about your experience right now.

 GUT CHECK:
WHAT MAKES YOU FEEL FULLY ALIVE?

Please take a moment, just one moment, and jot down three ways you feel fully alive. Refer to the examples on the previous page for hints. Use the lines below or write them in your journal:

1. Arriving at the peak of a challenging hike.
2. Thinking about a creative project.
3. Engaging debate / conversation on something I've learned about.

Try this every day for a month. Before closing your eyes at night, recall three moments or three ways you felt fully alive that day. Then list them in a journal or notebook. You don't need to explain why they made you feel alive; just list them. You'll soon learn to recognize moments of aliveness all the time.

Remember that feeling fully alive doesn't always mean feeling good or blissed-out. High-definition, high-voltage living is not always peaceful. Glimpses are snapshots of reality, your life exactly as it is in the moment — unfiltered. The more you get to know what makes you feel fully alive, the more often you'll experience high-definition, high-voltage living. This is precisely when you glimpse the space beyond your busy mind. This is where you meet your natural state.

Your Natural State

Your natural state is ordinary and always available to you. It's a state in which you're present, simply living in the moment. You experience this very normal and natural way of being when you show up in this moment, aware of your senses and surroundings. You don't need to improve anything to meet this state. You access it when you shift your attention from busy mind to the space that lies just beyond thinking. In a matter of a few breaths, you have the capacity to shift from distracted to present, from frazzled to focused, and from confused to crystal clear. When you show up in this moment, you meet your most authentic way of being you. This is your natural state.

When you show up in this moment, you meet your most authentic way of being you. This is your natural state.

PRIMER PRACTICE:
SKY GAZING

Sky gazing is a way to shift beyond your busy mind and settle into a space where you can glimpse your natural state. This relaxing practice allows you to feel what it's like to experience high-definition, high-voltage living. Do this practice when you can look out a window or, better yet, sit outside. It can be done day or night. Join me for a guided Sky Gazing practice on the Verge Mobile App.

1. Settle into your seat or lie down. Set your timer for at least five minutes.
2. Close your eyes and take three deep breaths.
3. Now, bring your attention to your exhalation. Don't strain to focus; just rest your attention on your exhalations.
4. Open your eyes and look at the sky. Rest your gaze softly on the wide open sky, not focused on any particular object.
5. With each exhalation, allow thoughts, distractions, and emotional tensions to gently release out of you into the vast sky. If a thought comes up, simply focus your attention on your next exhalation and allow the thought to pass. Repeat as often as necessary.
6. Allow yourself to be absorbed in looking at the sky, resting in the space inside of you, around you, and above you.
7. Notice your experience.
8. Continue until your timer goes off or, better yet, stay for as long as you like.

Glimpsing Your Natural State *Is* Being Fully Alive

Being fully alive is who you are beyond your stories, roles, and beliefs. Call it energy or awareness. In the context of this book, the words you adopt aren't important, as being alive is ultimately indefinable and ever changing.

Don't let the terminology confuse you. Ultimately, being fully alive goes beyond definitions — it must be directly experienced. What I'm here to point out to you is how your busy mind operates, so that you can recognize moments when you're not living from your busy mind, moments when you're living from your natural state. And it's there, in the space beyond thoughts, doubt, and fear, where you feel fully alive.

I've had thousands of my own such glimpses of being fully alive not only standing on my yoga mat or on a mountaintop, but also with my family, in my car, and even while writing this book. You've had them too; you simply haven't been paying attention to them — yet.

Being fully alive isn't a feeling that just happens when you're at the beach or even in the middle of a crisis. It's a direct experience of high-definition, high-voltage living. It recharges you in ways that you can now only imagine. Some days you may feel it faintly, and other days it will light you up. Don't try to do anything special. You are already fully alive. You are already on the verge. Just take a breath, keep reading, relax, and enjoy.

> Being fully alive goes beyond definitions — it must be directly experienced.

PART II

YOUR
NATURAL STATE

CHAPTER FOUR

Clear Mind

E very Sunday in the fall, for the past twelve years, I've been training the Villanova University football team. As a mental strength coach, I move ninety young men through a yoga and meditation session. The purpose is to strengthen their capacity to stay composed under the fire of competition — to be mentally stronger when physically challenged. I train them to be mentally steady and emotionally stable. Thankfully, they listen to me. The Villanova Wildcats know what a team that's strong, stable, and clear can achieve — out of the past twelve seasons the Wildcats have been in the playoffs ten times, and in 2009 they won the FCS National Championship.

Mental strength is your capacity to show up in this moment and pay attention to what's happening. It's your ability to live on the verge. Are you actively engaged in reading these words or passively paying attention? Can you bring your attention back to this word? This is showing up, and when you do so, you're operating at full strength. You're clearer, wiser, more aware, and more compassionate. Everything you do you do better when you show up in this moment. You have more energy. You have more confidence. You are on the verge.

> Mental strength is your capacity to show up in this moment and pay attention to what's happening. It's your ability to live on the verge.

If you're passive or distracted, you're in a weakened mental state. It's that simple. If you're foggy or dulled, sort of right here and out there at the same time, you're less sharp and not at full strength or full capacity. You cannot be both on the verge and distracted in the same moment. You cannot be in your busy mind and show up and shine.

Welcome to Your Busy Mind

When you're distracted, your mind is busy hanging out in the past, in the future, in your stories. It's somewhere else — and in a weakened state. When you're distracted, your mind and body aren't working together. They're not communicating. They're not synchronized. You're not even experiencing what's happening in your body — you are somewhere else. You feel disconnected, off balance, or out of sorts. When you are distracted, mistakes happen.

Shift beyond your busy mind, however, and you arrive in this moment fully. When you show up in the now, your senses light up and your instincts are razor sharp. You experience the world in high definition. You feel crystal clear and fiercely focused. Your mind and body connect. They work together. They synchronize. You connect to your senses and glimpse your natural state. Step beyond your busy mind, and you're clear and confident — you are on the verge.

When you show up in the now, your senses light up and your instincts are razor sharp.

A few years ago, I was watching an NFL playoff game that came down to a field goal with less than a minute to play. As I observed the kicker walk onto the field toward the football, I commented to my family, "He's not going to make the field goal. Look at his eyes. See them shifting? You can feel his doubt." His body language transmitted his nervous tension; he was distracted, not tuned in to the moment, and definitely not on the verge. Yes, he missed the goal, and his team lost the game.

Traits of Your Busy Mind

Have you ever tried to stop your mind from thinking? It's not so easy, huh? The truth is that thinking is what your mind is meant to do! Your mind produces thoughts, just as your ears hear sounds and your eyes see your surroundings. Also, thinking isn't a bad thing; it's just that we're preoccupied and often obsessed with it. Our thoughts rule our lives. We believe that what we think is actually the way things are, that our thoughts perfectly reflect our reality. As a result, we become attached to our stories and end up engrossed in and even imprisoned by what we're thinking.

Your busy mind is made up of a mix of thoughts, emotions, doubts, and fears (along with various other thought patterns). By the way, it is the same for everyone. In our society of more and better, our minds operate with constant mental noise: planning, judging, analyzing, commenting, remembering, forecasting, and so on. You don't realize how much your busyness controls your day until you collapse on your bed at night.

Shifting beyond your busy mind doesn't mean you stop thinking, but it does change your relationship to thinking. Your thoughts and emotions stop ruling your world, and you learn to trust your direct experiences.

Shifting beyond your busy mind doesn't mean you stop thinking, but it does change your relationship to thinking.

Let me say that again in a slightly different way. You move from being led around town by your busy mind to trusting your direct experience, your firsthand knowledge, of the moment to inform you of what is real and true. That is not to say that you're going to disregard your thoughts and emotions; you're simply changing your relationship to thoughts and emotions by recognizing that they don't always clearly reflect reality.

In order to understand how your thoughts and emotions may be ruling your world, it is essential to get to know your busy mind. Some common traits of the busy mind are sloppy brain, being crazy busy, being on autopilot, information overload, and overthinking. Let's look at them more closely.

Sloppy Brain

I call my busy mind my "sloppy brain" when I'm distracted and feel clumsy and out of sorts. Let's face it, sloppy brain happens to all of us. Recently I went to work with my slippers on. No joke! Luckily, as a yoga teacher, I spend most of my workday barefoot, but that still didn't protect me from the loving abuse I took from colleagues and students. I see examples of sloppy brain on the highway, in the grocery store — everywhere. Too many of us are sloppy in how we show up in our day-to-day lives. This isn't a judgment, just a fact.

The distracted, sloppy busy mind is in a weakened state. It speeds through life and doesn't slow down to take even a few seconds to tell you to, say, mindfully place your phone and keys in the same place, set your teacup away from your laptop, or notice the stop sign in front of you.

Crazy Busy

"Crazy busy" has become a common phrase and an accepted way to live. We're so addicted to getting things done that we're oblivious to what's really happening around us. Just look around any public area, and you'll see most people looking at their phones while waiting in line, walking, or even talking with others.

When you're in "crazy busy" mode, you're not really focused

on what you're doing or whom you're with. Your mind is too busy processing stuff to do, daily activities, and places to be. Being "crazy busy" can make you feel as though your world is spinning out of control and there's no end in sight. It's not just you. It's most of us. How often have you greeted friends and boasted about being "crazy busy"? The bottom line is that you cannot feel awake and fully alive when your mind is "crazy busy."

Autopilot

Many of your daily activities are repetitive, like brushing your teeth, checking emails, taking a shower. The thoughts streaming through your mind tend to be repetitive as well. Many of today's thoughts were yesterday's thoughts — they keep replaying in your head. For example, you might think, "I have to go to the post office," over and over for two days straight until you actually go to the post office. The script for autopilot is often a thought loop that keeps running in your head: "I need to lose weight," "I need to make more money," "I should clean my closet," and so on. When you're on autopilot, you think the same thoughts over and over without being aware of it. Living on autopilot is exhausting and will leave you feeling drained at the end of the day.

I observe autopilot in action all the time. Students rush through the doors, throw down their yoga mats, and lie down for a moment before class to "quiet their minds." I'll see them glance around for their cell phones (which are not allowed in the yoga room) or look for someone to talk to (no talking before class either), unaware of these mental habits and tendencies, especially the need to be constantly entertained.

Information Overload

Everywhere we look, we are surrounded by information to process and choices to make. Experts tell us to do this, buy that, and

eat this. Bombarded by advertisements, news, emails, and sense-
less posts on social media, our mental hard drives become over-
loaded, inefficient, and sluggish. Every day, your busy mind tries
to absorb and remember the onslaught of information coming
across your mental screen. In our overstimulated society, living in
the busy mind can lead to exhaustion and fatigue, chronic stress,
and even depression.

Overthinking

Last, overthinking is a major cause of chronic stress in our highly
demanding culture. On any given day, you experience thousands
of repetitive thoughts, many of which are tainted with judgment
and anxiety. Too much planning, worrying, and replaying these
loops is exhausting. Incessant thinking creates tension and robs us
of peace. Although thinking is useful, overthinking is draining.
Although stress is necessary to flourish at times, chronic mental
stress causes chronic physical stress, which is harmful to your
health.

Get to Know Your Busy Mind

Sloppy brain, being crazy busy, being on autopilot, information
overload, and overthinking leave you with little time to be in the
moment and little space to show up and shine. Your muddled busy
mind becomes the filtered, blurry lens through which you experience life.

Do you live with a busy mind? Are you distracted much of
the time? Welcome to the club! Take a deep breath and get excited, because you're going to discover how to consistently slow
down, settle down, and shift beyond your busy mind.

Let's first get to know what this busy mind of yours is so busy
doing.

◆ GUT CHECK:
YOUR BUSY MIND

Take a moment to answer these two questions either on the lines below or in your journal. Your answers will help you get to know your busy mind and how living from it affects your daily activities, relationships, and overall sense of well-being.

List three times during your day when you're most likely to be distracted, hurried, or anxious (for example, when you're driving, reading, answering emails, or eating):

1. _____

2. _____

3. _____

Off the top of your head, list three traits that describe your busy mind (for example, feeling overwhelmed, scattered, anxious, rushed, or drained):

1. _____

2. _____

3. _____

Your answers to these questions will offer you new opportunities throughout the day to become familiar with your busy mind. For example, if you tend to space out while driving, use driving as time to practice noticing your direct experience of driving. Turn off the news or music and notice everything around you. Notice the sky, the light on the trees, the noise around you, and how your body feels behind the wheel. Then notice when you forget to notice, when you drift back into your stream of thinking. This is how you train your mind to show up. You notice, notice, notice.

Becoming familiar with your busy mind and how it works is your first step toward understanding how to shift beyond it. You do this by getting to know how your mind operates with a practice known as *mindfulness*.

Mindfulness is your capacity to show up in this moment and be fully engaged from the level of mind, body, and heart. It's your ability to notice your firsthand, direct experience of what's happening — no matter if what's happening is good or not so good. To be mindful is to simply notice when you show up and when you don't, when you're on the verge and when you're not.

> Mindfulness is your capacity to show up in this moment and be fully engaged from the level of mind, body, and heart.

You become mindful when you notice that you're distracted. The moment you notice that you're not paying attention, you wake up — instantly! Noticing is enough, every time.

Noticing when you're passive wakes you up. Noticing distraction wakes you up. This is how you cultivate mindfulness. Notice. Notice. Notice. You can remember to notice by asking yourself the following question several times per hour: "Am I distracted or am I right here right now?"

Ask this question, and it interrupts your mind from whatever it was distracted by (a tense situation at work, the beach, ice cream) and brings you back to the moment (in front of a field goal, a crying child, or a traffic jam). In a second, you can shift from busy mind to clear mind. You pull yourself back into the moment. That's all there is to it. It's really a very simple, ordinary thing to do. That's mental strength training.

To practice mindfulness, show up in this moment, notice when you're pulled away by a distraction, and, without judging yourself, show up for the next moment. Do this again and again. Notice that your busy mind is undisciplined. Notice how easily you're distracted. Be prepared to notice a lot of distraction. Doing this over and over again — that is how you practice mindfulness.

Think of your mind as a muscle that becomes weak and atrophies when not used properly and becomes stronger and more stable when challenged to grow. In other words, your mind, if untrained, is weaker and likely to be easily distracted and flustered. Your mind, if disciplined, is stronger and likely to be focused. Imagine noticing as doing bicep curls for your mind. To build muscular strength, you need to either continually increase the repetition of bicep curls or add more weight over time. In the same way, you'll need to practice noticing and showing up more often or for longer stretches.

Mindfulness is your mental strength training.

Noticing is like doing a bicep curl. Mindfulness is your mental strength training.

PRIMER PRACTICE: DISTRACTED OR RIGHT HERE RIGHT NOW?

Read through the instructions first or listen to the guided practice on the Verge Mobile App. Commit to trying this right now. What do you have to lose? Perhaps just your busy mind!

1. Get settled in your chair.
2. Place your hand just beneath your navel, so you can feel the gentle rise and fall of your belly as you breathe. Take a breath in, and in your mind say, "Inhale." Pause after your inhalation, saying, "Pause." Breathe out slowly, saying, "Exhale." Pause after your exhalation, saying, "Pause." Repeat.
3. Continue to breathe this way, saying in your mind, "Inhale, pause, exhale, pause."
4. When you notice you've become distracted by thoughts or sensations (and you *will* become distracted), say in your mind, "Distracted."

5. Give yourself a mental high five for noticing.
6. Then immediately say in your mind, "Right here right now."
7. Place your attention back on your hand on your belly and on your next breath.

It's very simple. Identify what you're doing (inhale, pause, exhale, pause), notice distraction, give a mental high five, and actively bring your mind back to your breath — over and over again. This is your mental strength training.

The point of this Primer Practice is to get to know your untrained busy mind. Remember, your busy mind is not "bad"; thoughts actually create great stuff. If you let your busy mind rule your world, however, you'll miss opportunities to directly experience your life in high definition.

Am I distracted or right here right now? Ask yourself throughout your day, and notice how it interrupts your tendencies to overthink, be crazy busy, suffer from information overload, or operate on autopilot or with sloppy brain. This is how you shift from busy mind to clear mind.

Clear Mind: Your Natural Sense of Clarity

When you slip into the space beyond your thoughts and emotions, even for one moment, you immediately feel clear and alert. This is called waking up. Shifting from busy mind to clear mind, from distracted to right here and now *is* waking up — you show up in this moment in your naturally occurring state of clear mind. In the space of your clear mind, you are on the verge.

I run a few times per week. I run to clear my mind. I don't care how far I run, and I certainly no longer care about my pace. I run simply to breathe and move. Breathing and moving in rhythm shifts me from busy to clear fairly quickly. The steady motion of my body when synchronized with my breath settles my thoughts and calms my nervous system in a way few other activities do. Beyond my busy mind I glimpse my natural state of clear mind.

Compared to the stuffy, crowded feeling of your busy mind, shifting into your clear mind feels like a huge relief. It's as if a gust of sweet spring air sweeps through your mind. The mental fog dissipates, tension dissolves, and your senses come to life.

When you shift into a clearer state, you experience the world in high definition. The sky appears bluer, noises are crisper, smells are stronger, tastes are more flavorful, and your body surges with energy. Beyond your busy mind, you feel fully alive.

> When you shift into a clearer state, you experience the world in high definition.

Although I can't tell you exactly what glimpsing your clear mind will feel like for you, I will say that training your mind will help you find out for yourself. Research proves that mindfulness practices work. A committed, consistent practice can change the physiology of your brain so that you're more engaged and less distracted. Mental strength training improves the way your brain works, and with practice you live more often from your clear mind and less from busy mind.

The Snapshot below offers you a handful of ways to recognize your clear mind. Pocket a few and use them in both your practices and your daily life.

SNAPSHOT:
YOUR NATURAL STATE OF CLEAR MIND

Alert	Composed	Settled
Stable	Free	Open
Calm	At ease	Radiant
Strong	Spacious	Unhooked
Present	Sharp	Awake

Besides feeling clear, shifting beyond your busy mind has many benefits. Accessing your clear mind offers you space and time to precisely assess situations, to stay open to the opinions of others, to regulate emotions, and to prepare appropriate responses in heated discussions. When you have glimpses of clear mind, you may find that you:

1. Speak genuinely and authentically
2. Connect more deeply with others
3. Feel relaxed
4. Are easier to be around
5. Rally others around your message and vision
6. Execute tasks with precision
7. Create with freedom and joy
8. Sense your intuition or inner direction
9. Know what to say and what to do

 GUT CHECK:
SLIPPING INTO CLEAR MIND

List three times when you most often feel mentally strong, stable, and clear (for example, when you're exercising, cooking, playing the guitar, or gardening):

1. _____

2. _____

3. _____

Busy mind or clear mind, distracted or engaged — you get to choose. You can choose to see the world through the muted and distorted lens of overthinking and "crazy busy" or experience life through the high-definition lens of your clear mind.

How do you choose? Notice this moment. Notice if you're distracted. When you notice, you shift beyond your busy mind.

When you notice, you glimpse the space beyond thought. You glimpse your natural state of clear mind. Notice and glimpse. Notice and glimpse. Remember, noticing is like doing bicep curls. This is mental strength training — small glimpses many times. Practice this consistently, and your thoughts and emotions will no longer rule your world. Instead, let your direct experience inform you of what is real and true in this moment.

Wake up, show up, and experience the world in high definition. Glimpse your natural state of clear mind, where you're not preoccupied with thinking and doing. Beyond your busy mind is exactly where you show up right here right now, and feel awake and fully alive. It's exactly where you live on the verge.

CHAPTER FIVE

Bright Body

For as long as I can remember, I've been fascinated with energy, how it moves and changes form. I've devoured books and teachings on the subject. I've used my mind and body as my laboratory to investigate how energy flows, where it gets stuck, and how to unblock, unfold, and unleash it.

I've been keenly aware of people's energy since I was a child. Although I didn't have the words to express my early awareness, I clearly remember sensing when those around me felt bright or dull, happy or sad. Of course, children are highly perceptive, so my sense of knowing was not unusual. However, my childlike curiosity went deeper. At a young age, I watched, even studied, adults as they waited in line at the store or sat on the train. I'd imagine what they were feeling.

Did they feel excited about their lives or were they struggling to get through the day? Were they positive or negative people? Fulfilled or discouraged? I pretended to consult with them about how they might feel better about their lives and what might help them feel physically brighter and mentally lighter. Little did I know, at six years old, I was reading people's energy and secretly giving them advice about how to feel more awake and alive. I've never told a soul this — until now.

Over the years, my curiosity about energy has not waned; in fact, it's grown into a profession. By teaching various movement disciplines, I've spent hours and hours with thousands of students without exchanging words. While guiding them into and out of Up Dogs and Down Dogs and many other yoga positions, I've developed a sensitivity for knowing if a person is feeling exhausted or empowered. In other words, I've spent my entire professional life communicating with people through the language of the body, the language of energy. I've dedicated my life to helping people manage their energy, and I want to help you do so too.

Live in the crowd and clutter of your busy mind, and you'll quickly feel drained. Shift beyond your busy mind, and you'll immediately feel a sense of relief. Slip into the space beyond your busy mind, and you vividly experience your senses. You glimpse your natural state from the perspective of your body, a sense of vitality called your *bright body*.

Like your clear mind, your bright body isn't a state to achieve. It's not anything you have to find; it's a shift in perspective, when you feel invigorated and strong. Glimpsing your naturally bright body is like plugging into an outlet and getting a jolt of high-voltage energy.

Live in the crowd and clutter of your busy mind, and you'll quickly feel drained. Shift beyond your busy mind, and you'll immediately feel a sense of relief.

High-Voltage Energy

Energy, the source of life moving through you and every other living animal and plant, cannot be created or destroyed, but it can change forms. It's experienced as power and is present wherever there's life. It's constantly shifting, rising, and falling. It directs every system in the body, sending messages through sensations, generating thoughts and emotions. Energy is the primal force of being alive.

Whether you feel energized or exhausted right now comes down to how energy flows through you. If you're jazzed about life, high-voltage energy seems to flow easily and abundantly. You feel radiant and empowered. If the chronic stress in your life has you feeling down and depleted, energy doesn't flow as smoothly or with as much power. You feel sluggish and discouraged. Your body feels anything but bright.

Circumstances arise every day that create barriers to energy flow. Many of these barriers are obvious: what you eat, how much you sleep, your activity level, and your environment. However, I'm not interested in telling you what to eat or drink or the best way to exercise. There's enough information out there about those topics.

I'm interested in helping you manage your energy by *doing* less and *being* more. I want to help you buzz at the highest level possible. I want to help you maneuver through your daily schedule, work, and social and family life with high-voltage energy. By shifting beyond incessant mental noise and exhausting emotional drama, you slip into the space of your natural state. We've already explored clear mind. Let's take a look at your bright body.

Bright Body: Your Natural Sense of Vitality

There are many obvious ways to maintain a high level of energy, such as daily physical activity, having rewarding work, eating healthy foods, getting plenty of sleep, and spending time in nature and with loved ones. There's also one simple way to open the channels of high-voltage energy in your life, all the time: shift beyond your busy mind and show up in this moment. Beyond your busy mind, you feel charged and ready to go — awake and fully alive.

If you want more energy, wake up and show up, right here and right now, in this moment, and this one, and now this one.

Get to know your bright body — it's the space in which you tap into your natural vitality.

Notice how you feel in the space beyond your busy mind. Glimpse the full, direct sensory experience of being on the verge, of plugging into your high-voltage energy. Get to know your bright body — it's the space in which you tap into your natural vitality. This is one of my favorite Snapshots. Just reading the descriptions gets me going.

⊙ SNAPSHOT: BRIGHT BODY

Fueled	Bold	Curious
Energized	Joyful	Empowered
Excited	Confident	Strong
Engaged	Alert	Charged
Radiant	Enthusiastic	Passionate

Drama Drains, Focus Fuels

In today's culture of overthinking and overdoing, it's easy to feel depleted. If you're like me, spend twenty minutes surfing social media, and you'll feel the energy sucked out of you. Get emotionally involved in someone else's family issues, and you'll find yourself caught in the web of drama. Take something too personally at work or get yourself caught in the middle of a controversy, and you will be dragged down by drama.

Drama happens when you experience life through the distorted lens of your busy mind. Being sucked into "he said, she said" leaves you feeling dull, drained, and at times annoyed. A small irritation or outburst can quickly sap your strength and make you feel less than bright. In short, *drama drains.*

I use the word "drama" to describe the destructive emotional traps you get caught in when you live from your busy mind. Whatever form it takes, drama will drain your energy. Take a look at the Snapshot of the ways drama may creep into your life, sucking the vitality right out of you.

 SNAPSHOT:
DRAMA-PRODUCING HABITS

Self-importance	Resentment	Worry
Needing to be right	Comparing	Self-degradation
	Whining	Belittling
Gossip	Regret	Ignoring
Judgment	Anger	Controlling
Jealousy	Expectation	Forcing

Spend too much time doing any of these, and you not only feel depleted but you also block your potential to feel fully alive. Get to know how drama operates in your busy mind. Stop the drama before it drains you. The Verge Practices and Strategies will help you recognize all the sneaky ways drama finds its way into your life.

As the Villanova football team approaches playoff time, I lean heavily on the idea that drama drains and focus fuels. I know these student athletes have loads of responsibility on their plate: schoolwork, practice, social life, and, you know — girls. College life, as you may remember, is nothing short of drama with a capital D.

> Get to know how drama operates in your busy mind. Stop the drama before it drains you.

As the playoffs approach, I coach them to actively pay attention to their energy. "Steer clear of drama. Don't create it, and don't get sucked into it," I tell them over and over. Nothing good comes of drama; it's a recipe for feeling exhausted and exasperated — on the field and off.

You can get sucked into drama just as easily as these college football players. Spend an hour, or even a day, absorbed in the ending stages of a romantic relationship, and you'll feel unsettled, exhausted, and out of sorts. Old grudges can be the worst culprits. Negative self-talk, gossip, and jealousy can make your world feel dismal, dull, and at times "sticky."

Sticky is how drama feels. Have you ever noticed that situations get sticky when you try to make life work out in your favor? Or when you try to fix people or avoid uncomfortable conversations? Sticky happens when you try to force the world to move — for you. When you act out of self-interest, more often than not you'll piss someone off, leaving you and the other person feeling drained and depleted.

That life gets sticky sometimes has nothing to do with you. Employees quit their jobs, people lie to their partners, and life gets pretty messy, right? Drama is created not because of what is happening, but how you relate to what is happening. If you remain clear and steady in the midst of the stickiness of life, you'll feel just like Teflon — someone else's drama will just slide right off of you.

I'm not telling you to ignore or run away from life. I'm saying that you don't need to be ruled by your emotions or the unpredictable emotions of others. Get to know your busy mind, so that you can shift your perspective beyond it. Get to know how you feel in sticky situations. Pay attention to how drama drains. Take a look at this Snapshot. Do you recognize any adjectives that describe some of the ways you feel when caught in drama?

> I'm not telling you to ignore or run away from life. I'm saying that you don't need to be ruled by your emotions or the unpredictable emotions of others.

SNAPSHOT:
FEELING STICKY .

Forgetful	Lazy	Annoyed
Irritated	Prickly	Unhappy
Sluggish	Fuzzy	Unclean
Clumsy	Weak	Unsettled
Heavy	Diminished	Cloudy

The first step toward limiting the draining effect of drama on your energy is to become aware of the environments in which you are most susceptible to getting caught in or creating it. Let's take a look.

GUT CHECK:
STICKY SITUATIONS AND STICKY PEOPLE

List three people or situations that create drama and leave you feeling sticky (for example, listening to your coworker whine, fighting traffic, or reminding your son to complete college applications):

1. _____

2. _____

3. _____

Hold on to these important clues for now; we'll come back to them later when you practice *Let It Go, Let It Be*. For now, pay active attention to other drama-filled moments and sticky situations and people who seem to drain your energy. Try not to judge them as good or bad. Simply become aware of them. Keeping a list can help you to recognize patterns of the ways that drama drains you.

As a mother of two college-age daughters, I'm all too familiar with the consequences of riding an emotional roller coaster for too long. As typical young adults, my girls are filled to the brim with both enthusiasm for life and dread-filled drama. They ride the emotional roller coaster like nobody's business. In fact, when either of them calls me from school, I've learned to pause and take a deep breath, so I can prepare myself for what might come. I'm never sure if I'm going to be greeted by joy and enthusiasm or heartbreak and tears.

Hang around young adults for a day or so, and you'll quickly realize that flying through life propelled by the whims of emotions and bouncing from one sticky situation to the next is an exhausting way to live. Luckily, most people grow out of that extreme, high-speed, loop-de-loop energy as they age. However, you may still find yourself on an emotional roller coaster — feeling high in the morning and low by the afternoon or just the opposite, bummed out in the morning and ready to rock by evening. I know you'd agree, this is an ineffective and inefficient use of your energy.

Cynthia's Roller-Coaster Ride

To more fully understand the flow of energy and how it's so easily blocked by drama, let's take a peek at a day in the life of Cynthia, a young single mother and student of mine. She told me of a particular spring morning when she woke up feeling supercharged about life. As she described it, she was "all high voltage." She sprang out of bed, sang in the shower, and joyfully packed her children's lunch. "It's going to be a great day," she thought.

By mid-afternoon at work, Cynthia felt as though she'd been run over by a truck. Without an obvious reason, she felt exhausted. Other than a few issues — an overdue and still unfinished project for her children's school and her boyfriend's canceling dinner for that evening — it hadn't been a particularly stressful day. We deal with small stresses like those every day. No big deal, right? Let's face it, small inconveniences happen all the time. As we know, there are always balls to juggle and unexpected issues to deal with. But Cynthia couldn't let go.

As the morning had progressed, Cynthia kept getting distracted by worrying about the school project and the possible reasons why her boyfriend canceled dinner. The anxiety zapped her energy. She began talking out loud to herself and hastily submitted a spreadsheet without checking it. No longer feeling sharp and enthusiastic, Cynthia hunched her shoulders as she pushed through the rest of her workday. She couldn't seem to shift herself out of the negative state. She got stuck in her busy mind.

On her way home she skipped the gym, drove past the grocery store she needed to go to, and barked at her kids when she walked through the door. Feeling overwhelmed and frustrated, Cynthia couldn't believe that just that morning she'd felt so energized and empowered. She'd gone from feeling bright to miserable, from feeling focused to fuzzy all in a matter of hours.

All in all, nothing terrible had happened to Cynthia. She just got caught in the web of drama and emotional turmoil in her busy mind. She started strong, but crashed and burned by midday. If Cynthia could have paused for a few minutes or even a few breaths to settle her thoughts and calm her nervous system, she might have been able to interrupt her downward spiral. Pausing to remember how energized and bright she had felt that morning could also have helped her to shift beyond the battlefield of her busy mind into the space where she would find some clarity and sensibility. Any kind of short break — going for a short walk or closing her eyes for five minutes — might have helped her shift perspective, show up for the rest of her workday, get to the gym, and be available to her kids.

Pause and Drop the Drama

You can interrupt a potentially destructive moment by pausing to sit still or to take a few breaths. You can disrupt an unhealthy pattern or unhelpful habit by doing the same. Your power is in your ability to pause. One simple pause can go a long way in shifting you beyond your busy mind.

GUT CHECK:
WHERE DO YOU GO TO REFUEL YOUR ENERGY?

In order to prepare for your next Primer Practice, list three places in the world where you feel most empowered and energized (for example, your bed, your backyard, or on top of a mountain). Be sure to pick really good answers, as they're going to come in handy:

1. _____

2. _____

3. _____

GUT CHECK:
WHAT DO YOU DO TO REFUEL YOUR ENERGY?

List three actions that empower and energize you (for example, skiing down a mountain, playing an instrument, or looking out at the ocean):

1. _____

2. _____

3. _____

The places and actions that charge you with energy are like your electrical outlets. They fuel you up and make you feel bright.

Keep these "go to" places or actions in your pocket. You'll use them in a moment.

 PRIMER PRACTICE:
REMEMBER THE VIEW

This Primer Practice is practical and easy to do. Give it a try now, and then also do it in your daily life. This practice can shift you from sticky and drained to bright and energized. Join me on the Verge Mobile App for an extended version of this Primer Practice. Let's begin.

1. Choose one of your "go to" places or actions from the previous two Gut Check exercises.
2. Take a seat, close your eyes, and take three long, deep breaths.
3. Bring this experience to your mind and pause.
4. Try to mentally re-create this experience with as much detail as possible. For example, remember how your body feels. What is your heart rate like? How do your muscles feel? Are you smiling, intensely focused, or peaceful and at ease? Place your full attention on re-creating this place or action. What do you smell, see, hear, or taste?
5. Resting in the quiet space of this particular view, allow your body and mind to absorb the moment. Notice your body and mind in this moment. How do you feel right here and right now?
6. Take note of any shift in perspective you feel.

Remember the view: This Primer Practice interrupts your tendency to get caught in drama and strengthens your connection to being bright.

I remember the view at least once every day. If I feel drama brewing (which I first sense as stirring in the pit of my stomach), I pause and remember one of my "go to" places or actions. Within a few cycles of breath and a few moments in silence, I feel brighter and more energized. This practice has helped me build trust in my natural state. I am confident that I don't have to succumb to habits of gossiping or judging. I can instead remember how empowered and energized I've felt in the past. This shifts my perspective in a matter of moments. My go-to places and actions are very ordinary. Here are a few:

- I live alongside Valley Forge National Park, a 3,000-acre piece of American history that consists mostly of wide-open fields. I can be found in the park almost every morning or evening. The spectacular expansive views never fail to clear my head and rejuvenate my body.
- Another go-to view for me is my shower — seriously. The sensation of hot water on my head clears and calms me as almost nothing else can. A shower can shift me from sticky to bright almost immediately.
- Finally, I go straight to the porch of the lake house in New Hampshire we rent for a week every summer. Remembering the view of the water and the mountains and the quiet serenity I always feel there can immediately shift my state.

There's a better way to live that goes beyond words — a way that only you can experience for yourself. Drop the drama before it drains you. Shift beyond your busy mind and remember the view. Remember what your bright body feels like and how charged you feel when high-voltage energy moves through your life. If you don't like what you're experiencing in any given moment, if feeling sticky or busy or anything else keeps you from feeling awake and alive, then know you have a choice — thankfully, you always have a choice.

Shift beyond your busy mind, beyond expectation, judgment, and the need to control, and you'll open the floodgate for high-voltage energy to surge through your life. Trust that there's power in the pause and that you can take a moment or two to shift beyond your busy mind and live from your naturally bright body. When you do, you'll light up the world with your high-voltage energy.

CHAPTER SIX

Open Heart

In March 2015, Cayman Naib, thirteen, a delightful and preco-
cious middle-schooler and the son of two of my dearest friends,
went missing. He walked out of his house on a foggy wintry night
in suburban Philadelphia. After a gut-wrenching few days of
searching for Cayman, we discovered he'd taken his own life just
a mere hundred yards from his home.

It was a life-changing week, one in which I learned what it
means to be available and open to life — just as it is. My husband
and I arrived soon after Cayman went missing, stayed close by
our friends as hundreds searched for their son, and stood by their
side during press conferences and memorials. We listened as they
recalled memories of their son's short life. We laughed and cried
with them every evening over food and wine.

During these precious days, I experienced a profound intimacy with life and death. What I learned in those tender moments
with my friends — while holding their hands as they waited for
news of their son, while holding space for them as they began
to grieve his death — is that living on the verge is not simply
about showing up in this moment, blissed-out, calm, clear, and
all that stuff. Living on the verge is about meeting life head-on
— right here and now — without hiding from the unfamiliar
or the uncomfortable. It's about being available in this moment

without feeling the need to control, fix, or impose your agenda and answers. Living on the verge is about being fearlessly open and sincere.

When your heart opens, you access your natural sense of confidence. It emerges when you embrace the moment fully — no matter what is happening. When you show up, available for life just as it is, you feel fully awake and alive.

Life is bursting with opportunities to be available and experience fully. Spontaneous sounds, smells, and scenes pop up everywhere. Some stop you in your tracks. Some even bring you to your knees. The sweet smell of lilacs, the cooing of a dove, or the tender text exchanges with your partner are all reminders that your life is meant to be experienced right now — not later when you have more money or more time — but right now. Shift beyond your busy mind often enough, and you build trust that you can embrace life fully — no matter what is happening. This is the confident nature of your open heart.

I stood by the side of my friends when they held a televised press conference about their missing son and made myself available for them. I stood by their side just waiting to offer a hug or a smile or to share a good cry. I found the courage to set aside my own fears and worries about Cayman and death in general to show up unconditionally for them. I was able to get out of my own way in order to fully embrace the unimaginable moment of anguish and intensity when Cayman's body was found.

I directly experienced the reality of this tragedy in the most intimate and vulnerable way — from my open heart. I felt alive in a way I can't describe. Those days are burned in my memory — in high definition. I'm so grateful I was able to show up and be available for those tender moments, moments that will be with me forever as some of the most vivid direct experiences of my life.

Embrace Life Fully — No Matter What

Sometimes life arrives wrapped up in pretty bows, with music playing and a sunset in the background, and sometimes it doesn't. There are moments of pure joy, not-so-ideal moments, and downright crappy moments. There's the good, the bad, and the ugly all wrapped up in one lifetime.

When life gets challenging, many people shut down. It's how we're conditioned. We throw up the walls to protect ourselves from feeling uncomfortable. When things fall apart, whether big or small, we run for cover, close the curtains, and hunker down for a nice long nap until the sun comes out again.

When life gets tough, we want out. We'll resist and ignore the unpleasant and do anything but embrace it. The truth is that uncomfortable and even painful moments are often so intertwined with brilliant shiny moments that shutting down to one experience causes you to shut down to them all. If you run away from the unpleasant experiences, you'll likely miss some pleasant ones along the way. Denying darkness only blocks your potential to experience brightness.

> If you want to directly experience being fully alive and intimately connected with the richness of your open heart, you'll need to embrace everything — not just the sweet moments — but every moment.

If you want to directly experience being fully alive and intimately connected with the richness of your open heart, you'll need to embrace everything — not just the sweet moments — but every moment. To experience the highest highs, you must be available for the lowest lows, to face stuff you're inclined to push away, avoid, or ignore.

Are You Showing Up or Shutting Down?

You cannot fully experience life if you push away, run away, or shut down. When you do so, you become unavailable. Instead of directly experiencing the world in high definition, you peek at it from behind the curtains of your busy mind. The practices you're learning here will help you recognize the difference between showing up and shutting down. You'll notice how you push away, avoid, or ignore painful feelings and sensations or those you'd rather not deal with.

Are you willing to participate in life fully — no matter what? If you're not answering with an emphatic *yes*, I highly recommend finding out why. Let's take a look at how doubt, fear, worry, and self-judgment may be getting in your way.

Doubt

Doubt is a sense of uncertainty or a lack of conviction, and it often shuts down our enthusiasm to embrace life fully. With information bombarding us 24/7, it's easy to latch on to a bit of news and run with it. For example, you can easily grab on to that one short article that says the benefits of meditating are inconclusive and, boom, you're done with meditation. Doubt is sneaky. When caught in doubt, you experience life through a filter of skepticism, indecision, and hesitancy. Doubt can easily convince you to run away and avoid an issue.

If you're not paying attention, you'll begin to also doubt your own direct experiences. You may even lose trust in your instincts to know what you need to be healthy and happy. Doubt keeps you trapped in your busy mind, where your tendency is to shut down or even hide from life instead of showing up and embracing life.

Fear

Everyone knows fear. It can save your life or keep you up all night. It arises when you anticipate danger or pain. Fear is one of the most powerful emotions we have. It's built into our DNA, an inherent instinct that acts as a warning system. Real fear has helped our species to survive; running back into the cave helped our ancestors avoid dangerous animals.

But there's another type of fear called "perceived fear." This fear is generated from your busy mind. There's the fear of scarcity, of not having people or things in your life, or of losing what you already have. There's the fear of missing out, the fear of the unknown, and the fear of death. These self-generated fears are constructed in your busy mind and are often described as False Evidence Appearing Real — FEAR.

Your body reacts the same way to a perceived fear as it does to a real one. During this physical response, your body releases stress hormones stimulating your "fight or flight" response. Instinctively this response prepares you to go into battle or flee. You become tense and rigid, not only physically but also mentally and emotionally. Let's look as some examples.

Real fear occurs when:

The car in front of you slams on its brakes.
The dish towel catches on fire while you're cooking.
Your toddler runs into the street.
A big spider lands on your arm.

Perceived fear occurs when:

You have thoughts of your neighbor's terrifying dog behind the fence.
You feel you might fall over a cliff, even though you're safely behind the guard rail.
You expect to get fired when your boss asks to meet with you.

Real fear keeps you alive. Perceived fear imprisons you in busy mind. Perceived fear cuts you off from your direct experience, making you unavailable for others. It mutes your confidence to experience deep intimacy and connection with life. It also blocks you from feeling fully alive.

Worry

Worry is a common strain of fear. It's manufactured in your busy mind and closes you off from your common sense. Worry is anxiety or uneasiness about potential outcomes. It's a sign that you're stuck in your busy mind. It manifests as stress, anxiety, nervousness, and even awkwardness; it makes you tense and distorts reality. Worry, the opposite of trust, also blocks you from receiving messages from your body.

Self-Judgment

Self-judgment is a critical view of who you are and what you're doing. It arises from constant comparison to others — what they look like, how much they appear to have, and even how happy they seem to be. In many ways, self-judgment is self-hatred. Sound harsh? Well, it is. Your negative self-talk pollutes every corner of your life. The quicker you recognize how harshly you judge yourself, the faster you can slay that dragon. Self-judgment cuts you off from living in high definition, and it crushes your high-voltage energy. Everything you see, taste, touch, feel, and hear will be distorted and muted when it's bathed in self-criticism. Eliminating this toxic habit is the true meaning of getting out of your own way. The Verge Strategy *Be Kind*, which you'll learn later on, will help you do so.

Become Familiar with Your Tendencies

Never underestimate the power of the deeply ingrained habits of doubt, fear, worry, and self-judgment, as they will shut you down and hold you back. These tendencies are like walls separating you from directly experiencing life. They block you from shifting beyond your busy mind and glimpsing your natural state, and they hinder your ability to be genuine and sincere.

I'm not suggesting you try to break these patterns. I'm not saying you can ever stop doubt, fear, worry, and self-judgment from arising. These are some of our most deeply rooted and in-stinctual human responses. However, I *am* suggesting that you become familiar with how they arise for you. Get to know your tendencies, and you can weaken their grip on your life. In other words, get to know how you shut down, and you'll discover how to show up.

> Get to know your tendencies, and you can weaken their grip on your life.

 GUT CHECK:
HOW DO YOU SHUT DOWN?

Take a moment to write down five ways that doubt, fear, self-judgment, and worry show up in your life (for example, you're impatient with your kids, you're addicted to checking emails, you feel bad about your body, or your neck is always tense):

1. _____
2. _____
3. _____
4. _____
5. _____

Doubt, fear, worry, and self-judgment are classic human traits that arise all the time. Look at them as hints or alerts as to why you're unavailable for the challenging moments of your life. When you get caught in your busy mind, let these deep-rooted patterns remind you to slow down, pause, and take a few breaths. By knowing how you shut down, you'll discover how to get out of your own way and open up to life fully.

Your Natural State of Open Heart:
A Sense of Confidence

An amazing thing happens when your mind and heart align. A tender confidence, a sweet, sincere trust in your instincts and insights, arises. Your natural state of open heart, along with clear mind and bright body, allows you to shift your perspective on how you are living and to be available more often to directly experience your life.

The experience of living with an open heart feels, to me, like standing tall with my arms stretched out wide and my palms facing up, ready to embrace the moment head-on. Being open-hearted means showing up for the good moments and the perhaps not-so-good moments. You get out of your own way and experience whatever life offers you right here and now. This is how to open up and be fully alive. This is living on the verge.

Start to notice ordinary moments of daily life when you feel open and available.

Start to notice ordinary moments of daily life when you feel open and available, those everyday opportunities when you are ready and willing to embrace life. For example:

Listening to your child tell a long convoluted story
Pausing to allow traffic to flow around you
Taking the time to consider someone else's point of view
Allowing your dog the time he needs to properly greet
    other dogs
Not being so quick to interject your opinion in a meeting
Giving your friend the extra time she needs to cry before
    giving advice

These examples may seem overly simplistic or even trite, but I assure you they're not. You cannot *try* to embrace life. You can, however, learn to recognize when you feel open and available and when you feel separate or closed off, when you show up and when you shut down. With practice, you'll learn to discern the difference between hiding in your busy mind and showing up to embrace everything.

**◆ GUT CHECK:
WHEN DO YOU OPEN UP AND EMBRACE LIFE?**

Write down five actions, places, or people that you already fully embrace. For example, I feel open when running in the park. I feel available when I read to my kids at night. I really appreciate the time I give myself to drink my coffee in the morning. List yours:

1. _____

2. _____

3. _____

4. _____

5. _____

I won't tell you what living from your open heart looks like or feels like, or when you're likely to show up and embrace life. To know your open heart, you must be willing to look at yourself in the mirror, up close and personal, and see what is shutting you down and holding you back. Take a look at this Snapshot.

 **SNAPSHOT:
YOUR OPEN HEART**

Availability	Appreciation	Fearlessness
Sincerity	Truthfulness	Curiosity
Compassion	Honesty	Authenticity
Patience	Joyfulness	Tenderness

Your heart is capable of being opened up in any moment. Most of the time, however, you're ruled by the chaos and clutter of your busy mind. Sometimes being open and available will occur in your life by chance, just as it did during my race; other times it may be more intentional, as it was with my friends last March. As with the clear mind and bright body, at first you experience your open heart through glimpses, and then you get to know it through practice.

 ### PRIMER PRACTICE:
BOX BREATHING

This practice synchronizes your mind and body by focusing on breathing rhythmically. It'll settle your thoughts and calm your nervous system, shifting you beyond your busy mind into the space where you can glimpse your natural sense of confidence. Try it for a few cycles or, better yet, a few minutes, or join me on the Verge Mobile App for a guided practice.

1. Sit with your feet on the floor and your hands palms down on your thighs. Try to sit upright in a relaxed yet alert posture.
2. Close your eyes.
3. Take a breath in through your nose for a count of four.
4. Hold your breath for a count of four.
5. Exhale out of your nose for a count of four.
6. Hold your breath for a count of four. (If the count of four feels too forced or too short, then simply change it. You don't want to feel as though you are holding your breath for too long.)
7. Notice how your belly expands as you breathe in and deflates as you breathe out. This is the work of your

diaphragm, your breathing muscle, that lengthens and contracts with every breath you take.

8. Repeat for six to eight cycles, or time your practice for at least two minutes.

This practice is meant to allow your nervous system to return to its natural state of rest and steadiness. Box Breathing will help you relax and settle down, even when you are anxious or stressed.

Trusting Life from Your Natural State

An amazing shift happens when you access your natural state of clear mind, bright body, and open heart. You begin to trust life. You let go of your need to control situations, and you give others more freedom. You settle down and start to allow life to unfold. This letting go is not about being passive. It's an active and powerful quality. Trust also promotes a sense of clarity and a deep knowing. It's not an intelligence that comes only from your mind; it's also a physical and emotional intelligence that emerges from your body.

Trust that you can be open and available to life under any circumstances, and you discover that you are already living on the verge. It's your most innate and instinctual way of being in the world. It's where you wake up and show up — and shine.

The Verge Practices that we're going to explore next will help you get to know your busy mind, how to shift beyond it, and how to glimpse your natural state every day. The point is to not just read about living fully, but to practice doing it, until living from your clear mind, bright body, and open heart becomes your normal way of moving and speaking in the world. This is when you'll embrace life and feel awake and fully alive every day.

PART III

VERGE PRACTICES

CHAPTER SEVEN

Awake and Fully Alive —
On Purpose

What you do every day matters. Your routines and habits set you in motion or bring you to a halt. They help you feel great or make you feel lousy. What you do on a daily basis has a cumulative effect on your life and has carried you to this very moment.

Do something every day that makes you feel happy and healthy, and you can call it a practice. Do something every day that shifts you beyond your busy mind and wakes you up to your direct experience of being fully alive, and we'll call it a Verge Practice.

Practices are powerful when they're done consistently. You can practice the piano or your golf swing. You can practice contemplative prayer, speaking the truth, or helping others. There are an infinite number of ways to practice.

You already have practices; you just may not label them as such — yet. You do stuff every day that makes you feel happier and healthier. Practices come in many different packages.

> You already have practices; you just may not label them as such — yet.

Here's an example of a seemingly insignificant practice. I set up my coffee pot in the evening, so that when I wake up early to write, my coffee is ready to be brewed. This simple routine really supports me. It's a small but significant treat. It's a way to be kind to myself, and it makes me feel happy.

Examples of other seemingly insignificant daily practices are:

Filling up the bird feeder in the morning to enjoy the birds throughout the day

Driving to work in silence, giving yourself space to mentally prepare for the day ahead

Walking around the block after dinner by yourself or with a family member to get your heart pumping

Preparing a healthy lunch to take to work, so that you aren't tempted to make unhealthy lunch choices

Lighting a candle every morning to evoke a sense of sacredness in your day

Reading a passage in a book of poetry or a spiritual text to relax you

Working on your hobby in the evening, even for fifteen minutes, to clear your mind and help you let go of the day

Getting up early to exercise and invigorate your body

Connecting with your children by listening to them review their day

There is a sense of calm about people who have crafted empowering daily practices. You may know a few folks like this, those who seem to stroll rather than sprint, like your gracious neighbor who cares for her flower garden every afternoon or your easygoing colleague who walks after lunch, rain or shine. How about your consistently kind friend who wakes before her family to sit in silence every morning?

Over the years, I've observed that poise and vitality seem to emanate from people who have established healthy daily practices. They somehow seem to be more productive, more engaged. They move through life with a calmness that makes them enjoyable to be around. They radiate a quality of excellence in the way they are living their lives. Though they may not realize it, these folks have learned ways to show up for their lives on a regular basis — they have discovered how to feel fully alive *on purpose.*

I've been so inspired by the positive effects of my practices and in observing how daily practices help others that I've dedicated my professional life to helping people establish and stay committed to their own. I'm excited to help you do the same by introducing you to some of my favorite practices — the Verge Practices.

Your Invitation to Be Fully Alive — On Purpose

The Verge Practices are not tricks to master; they are invitations to shift beyond your busy mind and directly experience being awake and fully alive — on purpose. These practices can shift your perspective from the crowded space of your busy mind to the open space just beyond it.

The Verge Practices are invitations to pause, look around, and look inside — to see life from a different perspective. They offer you space and time to get to know your busy mind and what it feels like to live in the space beyond it. Each Verge Practice is an invitation to become familiar with your naturally clear mind, bright body, and open heart. Each Verge Practice is an invitation to be awake and fully alive.

> The Verge Practices are not tricks to master; they are invitations to shift beyond your busy mind and directly experience being awake and fully alive — on purpose.

Imagine running on a treadmill while listening to music and watching the news. In need of a break, you jump off for a moment to catch your breath. Settling down, you notice your heart racing and muscles burning. You glance around the gym and take in the sights and sounds of the people and machines. During your brief pause, you notice that you feel connected — to your breath, to your body, and to the others in the gym. During the pause you experience a sense of aliveness, a visceral sense of coming home.

When your break is over, you get back on the treadmill, but leave your headphones off. Instead, you embrace all of the sensations in your body and continue to bask in the sights and sounds around you. You engage with what you're feeling and with what's happening around you. You feel awake and fully alive.

The Verge Practices are like taking a break from the treadmill and then getting back on with a different perspective. Each practice is a way to press the pause button during your busy life, so you can look directly at your busy mind and glimpse the space beyond it. When you return to life, you do so with a different perspective, from your natural state, where you are instinctively open, clear, and confident.

Verge Practices at a Glance

The Verge Practices are explained in the next four chapters and supported with guided practices on the Verge Mobile App. I highly recommend that you read each practice chapter before testing out the guided practices. With the expanded instructions provided in the practice chapters, you'll approach your new Verge Practices with a greater understanding, increasing your likelihood of staying committed and consistent for years to come.

The Primer Practices you've learned so far have been preparing your mind, or "priming the pump," for the expanded Verge Practices. The Primer Practices help you shift beyond your busy mind in a matter of a few breaths or a few minutes. They are not beginner practices; they are preliminary practices that you'll continue to do to settle your thoughts and calm your nervous system. As you'll see, the Primer Practices play an important role in the first Verge Practice.

Here's a sneak peak at the Verge Practices to give you a sense of where we're headed:

1. *Notice This Moment* sets the stage for all of the others. It is a set of mindfulness exercises, some of which you've already tested as Primer Practices, that will help you settle down, pause, and get to know your busy mind.

2. *Move My Body* is a practice that creates steadiness and stability in mind and body through breath and movement. By synchronizing or harmonizing your systems you'll experience spaciousness and a sense of vitality and well-being.

3. *Meet My Mind* introduces mindfulness meditation — training in calming and settling your mind and body, so you become familiar with your busy mind and the space beyond it.

4. *Notes to Self* presents three ways to converse with yourself — remind, ask, and intend. It is a unique practice to help you become both a coach and a friend to yourself by paying attention to your inner dialogue, interrupting your busy mind, and naming what matters most to you.

Before You Get Started

You'll be happy to know that the Verge Practices will fit into your daily routine right away. They don't require filling your day with more stuff to do or spending more money. You're overscheduled as it is and have likely purchased more fitness gadgets and organizing tools than you care to admit. The last thing you need is to try to set aside an extra two hours per day to practice. The bottom line is that if your practice is inconvenient, you're not going to do it. The Verge Practices are convenient and easy to understand.

The Verge Practices are convenient and easy to understand.

For instance, the Verge Practice *Notice This Moment* might involve pausing upon waking up to take about five deep breaths, then at work to take, say, ten breaths, and then later on, at home, to practice deep breathing for five minutes or longer. *Notes to Self* could mean stopping yourself for a moment to ask, "What am I resisting?" during a tense conversation with your partner or co-worker.

These practices are also easy to implement. The point of the Verge Practices is not to add more pressure to your schedule, but to show you how to recognize where you get distracted and stuck in drama and how to shift beyond your busy mind and glimpse your clear mind, bright body, and open heart.

Verge Practice Support

Throughout the next few chapters I'll coach you on how to really commit to practice. Staying consistent and having the right attitudes are essential to really gain the benefits of the Verge Practices. I'll say it again and again: stay consistent and adopt supportive attitudes.

Consistency Is Key

I'm not proposing that you do every practice every day. I use the term "daily" loosely to simply mean "consistently." My intention is not to stress you out and add more items to your already overpacked to-do list. It's to help you understand the transformative momentum that is generated by consistent actions. The goal is to be steady and consistent, not a slave to your schedule of practices.

I have practices that I do daily, such as meditation, journaling, and some type of physical activity, and I have practices that I do several times per week, such as yoga or strength training. I suggest you take your practice schedule lightly, because overcommitting is a sure path to failure, and believe me, I've learned that the hard way. Here's my take on what works.

Start small, stay steady, and build from there: Although the Verge Practices are straightforward and easy to do, they take commitment to master and time to develop. When you're getting started, it can be challenging to stay consistent with an unfamiliar routine. You may even feel clumsy. Success happens when you start small and stay steady. You'll build a strong foundation from which you can deepen and expand your practice.

> Start small, stay steady, and build from there.

In other words, it's better to devote some time to Verge Practices every day — even if it's just a little bit — than none at all. For example, sit quietly in meditation for five minutes, and do it every day until you can build to ten minutes. The same goes for moving your body and every other daily practice.

Timing is everything: In order to stay consistent, you will need an overall practice that works with your schedule, which I'm sure is a busy one. At first, it may be helpful to mark your individual practices on a calendar. An online calendar makes it really easy. Color-code your daily practices to make things fun. Synchronize your calendar with your phone to receive notifications. Download the Verge Mobile App for customizable practice alerts that will sync with your devices and online calendars.

Overuse of technology can leave us feeling as frazzled as our busy minds do. It can, on the other hand, be used wisely. Used mindfully, your devices can be extremely helpful in keeping you on track with your practices. Whatever works for you is what's right for you. We're all wired differently, so don't force yourself to use technology if it is going to cause you more stress.

Stay flexible: Life happens. Kids get sick. Snowstorms create havoc in your work schedule. As you become consistent in your practices, you'll find ways to maneuver around the changes in your schedule. You'll learn to shift this and that to make sure you practice, or you may even decide to skip practice that day. As you deepen your commitment to your practice, you actually become more flexible and less rigid. If you can't get to the gym one day because of a bad head cold, it doesn't become a huge problem.

Remember the "why": Having clear intentions of what you're doing and why is like walking around with a compass in hand, directing you toward your true north. Remembering why you're committed to your practices can be of great support in staying consistent. It's helpful to keep a list of the ways your practices support you in living on the verge every day. Here are a few to get you started. The Verge Practices can help you:

- Shift beyond your busy mind
- Show up in this moment
- Recognize direct experiences
- Become familiar with how your mind operates
- Glimpse your natural state of clear mind, bright body, and open heart
- Experience being awake and fully alive
- Drop your drama
- Embrace life fully
- Recognize when you're resisting
- Be kind to yourself and others
- Experience the world in high definition
- Access high-voltage energy

Keep building momentum: Like the process of building strength in your body, the more you practice, the more skilled you become. As your practice becomes a routine in your life, it will inspire you to stay committed. You keep practicing because your practice empowers and energizes you. This momentum becomes your "why" and your fuel to keep practicing.

Consistent practices build momentum, and momentum builds on itself. At some point, your Verge Practices will become what you do all the time without thinking about it, just as with your regular practices of making an afternoon cup of tea, walking around the block, or throwing the ball around with your dog.

The Right Attitudes

You can also support your commitment to practice by adopting the right attitudes right from the start. Practice attitudes are reminders to stay with your practices. Think of each attitude as a coach standing on the sidelines encouraging and inspiring you. The following attitudes can help support you in staying committed to your practices.

> Think of each attitude as a coach standing on the sidelines encouraging and inspiring you.

Keep it light: There is no better way to fail at anything than to beat yourself up about not doing it or doing it poorly. There's nothing more important than being gentle with yourself as you practice. Also, a little humor goes a long way, and having a good ol' laugh at yourself every once in a while keeps your heart open and light. Being as kind to and supportive of yourself as you would be with a child or a good friend is a great way to stay in your practices.

Drop all expectations: Dropping expectations for how you think your practice should feel opens up the door to experiencing what you are meant to feel right now. Allow your practice to unfold one day at a time. You will be amazed at what emerges.

Let go of perfection: It's called practice, not perfect. In fact, there is nothing to perfect with your practices. They'll continue to change and evolve. Learn to relax and enjoy the ride. In fact, the more you can enjoy being a beginner, the fresher your practices will remain.

Don't judge: It's much easier to read about this attitude than it is to execute it. Judging is a deeply rooted human tendency. Unfortunately, it's also a destructive one. Your practices are a great time to practice not judging! Allow yourself to mess up in your practice. Let yourself drop the ball. If you fall asleep in meditation, just open your eyes and try again. If you forget to pause and breathe before screaming at your child, put your hand on your heart and then give your kid a hug.

Acknowledge yourself: You may find it awkward at first to call your evening walk around the block a practice. But if you look at the benefits of your walk, such as getting some fresh air, connecting with your neighbors, and getting the kinks out from sitting all day, you'll give this simple routine the power it deserves. Acknowledge that walking around the block every evening can make you feel energized. Taking care of your well-being is a big deal. Feeling awake and fully alive is a *really* big deal!

Finally, each practice chapter begins with an At-a-Glance page summarizing the Verge Practice. You can bookmark these pages for easy future reference. I'll also support you with guided practices online. So let's do this — let's dive into our first Verge Practice, *Notice This Moment*, and start being awake and fully alive — on purpose.

CHAPTER EIGHT

Notice This Moment

At a Glance: Verge Practice #1

Purpose   *Notice This Moment* is a toolbox of practices offering you different ways of practicing mindfulness for different situations. The Primer Practices, those you've already learned and those coming up, are all included in this toolbox. *Notice This Moment* will help you settle down, pause, and get to know your busy mind.

Benefits   Noticing strengthens your capacity to be mindful, pay attention, and glimpse your natural state more often. It also can reduce stress and help you experience life more fully. This Verge Practice is the foundation for the other practices. It trains you to settle down, show up, and live on the verge.

How-To Primer Practices:

Stop, Take Five, Experience (p. 9)	Remember the View (p. 59)
	Box Breathing (p. 72)
Wake-Up Call (p. 18)	Counting Breath (p. 90)
Sky Gazing (p. 30)	Coming Home (p. 185)
Distracted or Right Here Right Now? (p. 43)	Body Scan (p. 198)

Mindfulness Reminder: No Speed, No Struggle (p. 91)

Online and on the Verge Mobile App: Guided practices for all Primer Practices are available on the Verge Mobile App.

As a figure skater, I quickly learned the cause-and-effect relationship between being either distracted or engaged. It was the difference between landing a double lutz and falling on my ass. When I showed up in the moment for a spin or a jump, I was transformed into an elegant example of strength and grace. Caught in a web of doubt or fear, for even a second or two, I crumbled into a jumble of arms and legs. From a young age, I knew the visceral difference between how I felt when I skated while focused and how I skated while doubting my ability. As any athlete knows, being focused, or "in the zone," is the stuff champions are made of. Training to notice when you're distracted, or not "in the zone," is the practice of mindfulness.

Notice This Moment is a set of mindfulness practices, or what I like to call mental strength training. Like any other training, you don't do it just once. The practice involves noticing this moment, and this moment, and this moment.

Mindfulness: Mental Strength Training

Mindfulness, as you know, strengthens your capacity to be aware of what's happening, to actively pay attention — on purpose. Our first Verge Practice, *Notice This Moment*, is training to catch yourself when you're not actively paying attention, when you drift away into busy mind, or when you're dull or foggy. This practice is a way of getting better at noticing when you're not aware. Over and over you notice if you're pulled away by thoughts. When you notice distraction, you immediately shift your perspective from passive to active, from busy mind to clear mind. This happens to you all day long — you wake up to what your mind is doing in short bursts here and there.

A Division 1 basketball player came to me because he was struggling with his free throws. Playing on a nationally ranked team in front of large crowds and often on national television had thwarted his ability to stay calm and cool on the foul line. He felt distracted and on edge and needed a tool to help him settle down. He agreed to try an exercise using a repeated phrase to help him become present and stay calm before shooting free throws. "Fierce focus" became the phrase he repeated as he stepped up to the line. His commitment to this simple practice paid off quickly as he learned to focus, improved his free-throw percentage, secured his starting position, and helped his team reach the NCAA Final Four that season.

> This practice is a way of getting better at noticing when you're not aware.

Champions are crowned because of their ability to consistently notice busy mind and shift into clear mind in key moments, whether on a sports field, in a boardroom, or at a recording studio. Like the basketball player who learned to repeat "Fierce focus" before free throws, you can strengthen your capacity to notice and shift, notice and shift, over and over.

Verge Practice: *Notice This Moment*

Notice This Moment is a toolbox of practices offering you different ways of practicing mindfulness for different situations. The Primer Practices you've already learned are included in your toolbox:

Stop, Take Five, Experience (p. 9)
Wake-Up Call (p. 18)

Sky Gazing (p. 30)
Distracted or Right Here Right Now? (p. 43)
Remember the View (p. 59)
Box Breathing (p. 72)

You will also learn a new Primer Practice called Counting Breath and a Mindfulness Reminder called No Speed, No Struggle. Two more Primer Practices, Coming Home (p. 185) and Body Scan (p. 198), will follow in later chapters. Just as you use different pieces of equipment at the gym, the practices in *Notice This Moment* train your mind, each from a slightly different angle.

Remember, the Primer Practices are designed to get you out of your busy mind, even if just for a moment or two. They help to interrupt distraction or drama and offer you a glimpse of the space beyond thinking.

Now let's learn two additional practices to add to your mindfulness toolbox.

PRIMER PRACTICE: COUNTING BREATH

Another practice to add to your toolbox is called Counting Breath. Although it's longer than your other Primer Practices, it's equally as simple and can be done anywhere. You can begin to practice right now.

1. Count down slowly from ten to zero. With each number, take one complete breath, inhaling and exhaling. For example, breathe in deeply saying "ten" to yourself. Breathe out slowly saying "ten." On your next in-breath, say "nine," and so on. When you reach zero, you should feel more relaxed.

2. Repeat this exercise several times for five to fifteen minutes.

3. If you find yourself distracted while counting, bring your-
    self back to ten and start over. It's okay, we all get dis-
    tracted, which is exactly why we are training our mind. Do
    this patiently and without judgment, and you will build the
    confidence to stick with this practice.

Monica, a stay-at-home mom of young children, told me that
she uses the Counting Breath exercise every afternoon as she
waits in the car line to pick up her children at preschool. She pur-
posefully arrives early and uses ten minutes of quiet time in the
car to settle her mind and to prepare for the busy evening ahead
with her kids.

This exercise is available to you whenever and wherever you
can remember to do it — on the train, in line at the store, or while
your emails are downloading. Take a moment now to try it on
your own or listen to the guided practice Counting Breath on the
Verge Mobile App.

Mindfulness Reminder: No Speed, No Struggle

There is an Italian saying that goes, *Chi va piano, va sano, va lontano.*
Chi va forte, va alla morte. Loosely translated, it means, "He who
moves slowly, moves peacefully and moves far. He who moves
too quickly goes right to his death!" My Italian grandmother, or
nonna, often preached this Italian proverb and emphasized the
morte by dramatically waving her hands in the air. "What's the
big rush?" she would ask in her heavy accent. "*Piano, piano*" —
"Slowly, slowly" — she mumbled to herself as I raced in and out
of the house.

When you move slowly and mindfully in your life, you experience less stress and less suffering. When there is no speed, there
is no struggle. In other words, trying to fly through your day, multitasking all the way, causes mishaps, oversights, and, well, more
stress and suffering. *No speed, no struggle*, I remind myself 24/7.

Now, thirty years later, I understand that my nonna taught me how to be mindful. She knew that if I could slow down physically, I would also slow down mentally, which would, in turn, cause me to struggle less and focus more and make me happier and ultimately more effective. *Grazie*, Nonna.

There are many obvious ways to practice slowing down. Since this exercise is so easy to implement, many people dismiss it. Here are a couple of ways that you can slow down. Hint: You don't have to do them all today! Choose one or two for this week or this month and then commit to practicing. You can practice No Speed, No Struggle by *slowing down* how you:

Breathe

Drive

Walk

Talk

Eat

Write an email

Clean

Shop

Cook

A great exercise reminder is to put a sticky note that reads "No Speed, No Struggle" on your steering wheel. Or put it on your computer screen. You can also repeat to yourself "slow down" as you transition from place to place or you can say what I like say to myself, *"Piano, piano!"* (hand gestures optional).

The toolbox for *Notice This Moment* is designed to be simple, so you can quickly experience what it feels like to shift from distracted to fully engaged in a matter of moments.

The toolbox for *Notice This Moment* — the Primer Practices and the Mindfulness Reminder No Speed, No Struggle — is designed to be simple, so you can quickly experience what it feels like to shift from distracted to fully engaged in a matter of moments. Let's take a look at a few of the many benefits of mental strength training.

Benefits of *Notice This Moment*

Millions of people have sought out instruction in mindfulness practices such as meditation, yoga, tai chi, and qi gong. Research has uncovered the benefits of these practices, and most of the results are extraordinarily positive. Mindfulness works! There is so much to gain from committing to training your mind. Here are just a few of the many scientifically proven benefits that come your way. Mindfulness:

- Increases your ability to pay attention
- Settles your mind and creates a sense of spaciousness
- Reduces stress
- Cultivates patience with yourself and others
- Helps you enjoy doing "ordinary" activities
- Makes you calmer and less reactive or angry
- Reduces judgment about others
- Reduces resting heart rate
- Improves digestion
- Boosts working memory
- Increases focus
- Offers a sense of peace
- Reduces chronic tension in the body

Practice Support

In my years of teaching, I've found that the following tips, tricks, and strategies help create the strong inner support necessary to stay consistent and committed to training your mind.

Be Consistent

The practices in the toolbox for this Verge Practice are ordinary and obvious. You may need reminders to help you simply remember to practice. Since your breath is always there to pay attention to, you may overlook it or push it aside for later. Since your ability to notice where you are and what you're doing is always at your fingertips, you may take it for granted and disregard its importance. Over the years, I've collected a handful of tips that can help you *remember to remember*!

Phone reminders: I love my smartphone and use my alarm and reminder apps to remember my practices. I get a kick out of my reminders — they make me smile — and give my daughters another reason to roll their eyes at me! Keep your reminders light and playful; otherwise, they become just another thing to add to your to-do list, and you and I both know that there are already enough things on that list.

Sticky notes: If technology stresses you out, then put the reminders on sticky notes and place them on your steering wheel, refrigerator, and computer screen. "Slow down" is a perfect reminder for most of our daily activities.

Bells: Buddhist teacher Thich Nhat Hanh is a big proponent of using everyday occurrences as practice reminders. He suggests that the sound of a bell ringing can remind you to practice mindfulness. Bells can include the sounds made by your phone, appliances, computers, or alarms. Be warned that there are bells everywhere in our lives; you may find yourself practicing mindfulness all the time!

Red lights: Sitting at a red light is a perfect time to practice mindfulness. Focused breathing is particularly helpful when sitting at a light or in traffic or standing in line at a store.

Thresholds: Another well-known practice reminder is to pause whenever you enter a room or cross a threshold. Pause and take a deep breath as you walk into your home or enter a building. Paying attention to the transition of entering a new space is an effective way of becoming present.

The Right Attitudes

Don't forget to carry the right attitudes with you as you embark on your journey of training your mind. These reminders will help keep you light and curious in your practices.

Stay flexible: You're not always going to remember to slow down or to pay attention. Some days there will be more speed or distraction in your life.

Keep it light: Everyone got a laugh when I showed up at work with my slippers on. It was fun to joke around with teachers and students. If you can learn to laugh at your momentary mental lapses, you'll recover more quickly and perhaps be more mindful when moving through the rest of your day.

Let go of perfection: No one is perfectly mindful and there are no Olympics for mindfulness, so relax and let go of trying too hard. Developing consistent practices is much more important than striving to be perfect.

Be patient: Also, please be patient with yourself as you explore this stuff. Enjoy the ride, including detours and speed bumps. Trust that you already have everything you need to learn how to slow down, breathe deeply, and show up for your life.

Don't judge: By becoming more mindful, you will become more aware of your internal dialogue. Notice what you say to yourself. This is the first step in changing what you may find to be a harsh way of judging yourself. Becoming more mindful actually helps you cultivate a loving attitude toward yourself and others. Remember: judge less, love more.

Let go of what's not working: You may find that some of my suggested practices just don't work for you right now. This is not a problem and is exactly why I'm offering you a collection of Primer Practices to choose from. Focus on what works and let go of the rest. You may find yourself using only a few of the Primer Practices.

Be kind: Treat yourself with care and respect. Everyone gets distracted, and everyone says or does things unconsciously from time to time. What's important is that you keep practicing. I like to put my hand on my heart and smile when I act in an unmindful way. Making friends with yourself is an invaluable strategy to carry with you and one we'll explore more later.

Living on the Verge

Training yourself to wake up, show up, and shift beyond your busy mind is a lifelong practice. Noticing this moment, over and over, is like taking baby steps. Remember, start small, stay steady, and you'll build from there. You don't want to jump out of the gate too quickly, and taking on too much too fast will exhaust your willpower. You want to ease your way in slowly. Carry your *Notice This Moment* toolbox of Primer Practices in your pocket. Count your breaths and settle your mind anywhere, check in if you are distracted or engaged, and slow down the way you move through the world.

Recognize how easy it can be to implement these practices in your life and to start paying attention moment to moment. I encourage you to commit, right here, to showing up in this moment over and over again. Don't wait until later. Now is your time.

CHAPTER NINE

Move My Body

At a Glance: Verge Practice #2

Purpose By synchronizing mind and body through breath and movement, you access your naturally bright body. During this moving meditation, you light up your senses, get your blood pumping, and invigorate every cell in your body.

Benefits Moving and breathing in rhythm synchronizes your systems and elicits an empowering sense of vitality and well being.

How-To *Move My Body* includes any kind of movement, including cardio activities, holistic training, strength training, and lifestyle activities. The practice template will help you organize an ordinary activity so that it can be an opportunity to wake up, energize, and feel fully alive. The template includes:

- Set an intention
- Warm up
- Move in rhythm
- Challenge yourself
- Cool down
- Rest

Online and on the Verge Mobile App: *Move My Body Practice Timer*; *Mindful Movement* practice (video), *Beginner Yoga* practice (video); *Synchronizing Mind and Body* all-levels yoga practice (video).

My philosophy is if you need to solve a problem, go out for a walk. Get some fresh air and clear your mind, and you're likely to return home with your answer. Move and breathe in rhythm for a prolonged period of time, and you'll settle down.

Move your body, and you'll get out of your own way. Move your body in rhythm, and you'll calm your mind *and* your nervous system. Move your body, and you'll shift your perspective from busy to clear. You'll undoubtedly feel lighter and brighter.

I've instinctively known the importance of movement my entire life. Moving my body stirs stuff up and shakes things out in a way that nothing else can. A good walk cleans the cobwebs out. A well-paced run steam-cleans my soul. A wide-open stretch of road on my Rollerblades frees my spirit. A strong, steady yoga practice empowers me. I could go on.

Your mind and body communicate through your nervous system. When your body feels sluggish, so does your mind. When you mind is frazzled, so is your body. Energized body, energized mind. Calm body, calm mind.

Energized body, energized mind. Calm body, calm mind.

Your mind and body are always communicating; it's just that your circuits get jammed from time to time. Stuck in your busy mind, you ignore your body and the sensations firing at every moment. You get so entrenched in your distraction and drama that you forget there's a living, breathing body below your neck! You know when you're hungry, thirsty, tired, and need to find a bathroom, but for many the communication ends there — unless, of course, your body starts screaming at you.

Live in your busy mind, and you remain unaware of the messages sent to you through sensations arising from your body. Move your body, even in the simplest way, and you'll open up the lines of communication between your mind and body once again. Move your body by intentionally harmonizing the rhythms of your mind, heart, and nervous system, and the lines of communication become crystal clear and very powerful. We'll call this synchronizing mind and body.

Verge Practice: *Move My Body*

The second Verge Practice, *Move My Body*, is an invitation to move rhythmically and breathe deeply as a way to synchronize your mind and body. Moving in this intentional way helps you to shift beyond your busy mind and tune in to your subtle and not-so-subtle physical sensations. Instead of having you exercise simply to work out and burn calories, this Verge Practice encourages you to move in a way that not only gets your blood pumping and invigorates every cell in your body, but also shifts you from feeling busy and distracted to clear and bright.

Synchronizing mind and body through rhythmic movement aligns your heart rate, brain waves, and nervous system. It brings your systems into harmony. There is nothing extraordinary about synchronizing in this way. In fact it's very ordinary, and you've done it many times. In this practice, you're going to learn how to deliberately restore balance and alignment by focusing on rhythmic movement and breath.

This Verge Practice is about forming a deeper connection between your mind and body. It's about experiencing movement from

Move My Body is an invitation to move rhythmically and breathe deeply as a way to synchronize your mind and body.

a new vantage point as a way to feel awake and alive. Let's get started.

Movement Categories

I've been training people to move their bodies for more than thirty years and have come across every body type and fitness level possible. I've taught people with prosthetic limbs and those who are visually or aurally impaired. I've taught folks who are super-stiff and those who are hyper-flexible.

Movement is movement is movement, so please drop any negative dialogue about how you're not in the best shape or you're not training for a triathlon. It doesn't really matter. Please forget about your ideal weight or the fact that you can't run anymore because of your bum knee. It doesn't matter. If you can move your arms and legs in some capacity, then we're in business, and even if you can't, we'll find a solution.

This Verge Practice is less about what type of movement you're doing and more about using movement to establish a *rhythm*. It's the rhythm that is key. The rhythm will help you synchronize your mind and body. It will help you shift beyond your busy mind and feel your aliveness.

On any given day, you'll choose from four categories of movement, each with specific benefits. Pick the category that's going to serve you best on that day. I'm not asking you to adopt all of these categories. Choose those that suit your lifestyle:

- *Cardio activities* are those that get your heart pumping and metabolism burning. They include walking, running, biking, swimming, rowing, and much more. Since cardio exercises are rhythmic in nature, they're a perfect choice for synchronizing mind and body.
- Commonly called mind/body exercises, *holistic training*

includes yoga, qi gong, tai chi, other martial arts, and other alternative practices. These disciplines are centered on balancing energy through focused attention and are effective in synchronizing mind and body.

- *Strength training* uses resistance, or added weight, to build physical strength, anaerobic endurance, and size of skeletal muscles. The exercises include traditional weight training with free weights, resistance bands, or machines and body-weight training such as push-ups and sit-ups. They add an element of focus and challenge to your practice.

- *Lifestyle activities* is a broad category of moderately intensive physical activities that includes movement you perhaps never considered to be exercise, such as gardening, climbing the stairs, cleaning your house, and even playing with your kids. I'd also include throwing a ball with your dog, dancing, and sightseeing. There's an element of rhythm in most types of activities. Get curious, and you'll find the one that works for you!

 GUT CHECK:
HOW DO YOU MOVE YOUR BODY?

Look at what you're currently doing and choose a new way of moving your body to start working on in the near future.

Put a check mark next to those categories you currently do and circle those you do not:

Cardio activities
Holistic training
Strength training
Lifestyle activities

List your current top three physical activities or training methods (for example, salsa dancing, rock climbing, and walking):

1. _____

2. _____

3. _____

List one you would like to try in the next two months:

_____

Move My Body Practice Template

It's time to turn your workout or activities into opportunities to feel awake and fully alive. It's all in the template. Follow along.

The *Move My Body* template can be applied to most types of activities. You're likely doing a version of this already. It's designed to get you moving and breathing in rhythm, so that you synchronize your mind and body. Doing so transforms your workout into an opportunity to shift beyond your busy mind and glimpse your natural state. The *Move My Body* template is:

- Set an intention (five seconds)
- Warm up (five to ten minutes)
- Move in rhythm (ten to twenty minutes)
- Challenge yourself (fifteen to thirty minutes)
- Cool down (five to fifteen minutes)
- Rest (five to ten minutes)

Set an Intention

As you tie up your laces, strap on your helmet, or even pull on your gardening gloves, bring some purpose to your practice. Take a moment to set an intention by thinking about why you're doing what you're about to do. Say your intention out loud or to yourself, but just do it. Then repeat your intention three times.

Intentions set your purpose into motion. Your intention could look like one of the following (the italics are what you'd repeat three times):

I'm going to *pick up the pace* during my walk.
I'm going for a run to *clear my head*.
I intend to *relax and enjoy* my bike ride.
I'm going to *embrace what I can do* during my yoga practice instead of what I can't do.

An intention is a powerful declaration of your willingness to experience life fully. It supports you in waking up and showing up in this moment. It provides the gusto behind your workouts and can keep you motivated and focused. Strong intentions bring strong results. Weak or uninspired intentions offer you the same in return. You will learn more about the power of intention with the Verge Practice *Notes to Self* in Chapter 11.

Warm Up

Next you'll focus on matching your breathing rhythm with simple movement for a few minutes. This slow, dynamic warm-up gives you the time necessary to settle your mind and prepare your muscles. By moving rhythmically, such as doing a few slow laps in the pool or on the track, you begin to steady your brain activity, heart rate, and nervous system. Your warm-up begins the process of synchronizing your mind and body.

Move in Rhythm

After a few minutes to warm up, pick up your intensity but stay in rhythm by coordinating your breath and movement. This is easy to accomplish while walking, running, cycling, or any other type of movement that's repetitive. For example, in yoga, you inhale as you raise your arms overhead and exhale as you bow forward, and so on. While hiking, you may walk in a rhythm that matches your breathing pattern. If you have trouble doing this, then simply focus on your breathing for a few minutes without stressing about it. Eventually you'll find some sort of rhythm.

Moving in a steady rhythm while focusing on breathing is a moving meditation. It settles your frazzled or busy mind, shifting you into your calmer, spacious, and more natural way of being. Even after just a few minutes of rhythmic movement, you start to feel the rhythm and you feel in the flow. Rhythmic movement sets a meditative tone for your practice. You can call it a runner's high. I call it being fully alive.

Moving in a steady rhythm while focusing on breathing is a moving meditation.

Challenge Yourself

Now that you are warmed up and settled down, it's time to turn up the heat by adding some challenge. Over time your body gets used to moving in a certain way and at a given level. If you don't push your systems to work harder or for a longer period of time, you won't get stronger. Challenging your muscles and your heart is essential. During yoga class, for example, you may challenge yourself in arm-balancing poses, warriors, and planks. If your activity is more cardio-based, your challenge may include speed intervals or a longer duration. If you're weight training, then you add challenge by increasing the amount of weight or repetitions of a drill.

In my experience, most people either speed past the challenge portion of their workout or skip it all together. Honestly, going at the same speed on the treadmill for thirty minutes may get you sweaty, but it won't over time build stronger muscles or a stronger heart. Challenge your body by really pushing the boundaries of what you think you're capable of doing, and notice how awake and alive you feel.

Cool Down

The final cool-down is extremely important, because it's your opportunity to be aware of the space beyond your busy mind. Unfortunately, many of us have been programmed to rush through or skip the recovery lap or the final twist or hip stretch. Your cool-down can include slowing down the pace of your movement until you come to a standstill or sitting on the ground to stretch.

This is the perfect time to check in with your sensations. Notice the way your body is buzzing or tingling. Notice the way your skin feels. Notice the sweat, the sun, your breath, and your mind. Notice, notice, notice without having to put words to your experience. There's so much happening in your cool-down that to skip it is a shame.

Rest

Now you get to taste the sweet nectar of your practice. When all is said and done, take a few minutes to rest — as in lie down and do nothing. Allow some time in your schedule to rest. Do not skip this step; it's your prize for taking the time to move your body.

You have everything to gain in taking a few minutes of rest, and nothing to lose. Pausing to directly experience being awake and fully alive is the essence of living on the verge.

In yoga practice we call this time to rest *savasana*, commonly translated as "Corpse Pose." It's a time to let go and recognize the symphony of sensations flowing in you and around you. It's a time to notice your sense of mental clarity and emotional availability. Instead of calling it "Corpse Pose," I call it "Alive Pose"!

During this final rest you experience feeling calm and alert, awake and aware. You've shifted past your busy mind and see the world in high definition — through the lens of your clear mind. You feel recharged with high-voltage energy. You feel complete and connected — at least for this moment. This is how you synchronize your mind and body through rhythm and movement. Now you're ready to step back into your life and directly experience each moment from a clearer perspective.

Practice Examples

Looking back on my final college track race, I realize now how synchronizing my mind and body had led me to run the race of my life. On my slow warm-up, I set an intention to run my "personal best" and settled my mind with the slow rhythm of my prerace jog. During the race, I connected my breath with the pace of my legs, shifting me beyond my busy mind and into a space where time slowed and my mind cleared.

You can do this too. You can turn most physical activities into a moving meditation and synchronize your mind and body. Let's look at how the template applies to a half-hour walk outside. Using this model, you can intensify or modify your activity as needed.

Set an intention: Why are you walking? How do you want to feel afterward? Do you want to clear your head, flush out an issue at work, or simply increase your heart rate?

Warm up: Set your phone timer for a few minutes and begin walking slowly. Bring your full attention to your breath and say or just think, "Inhale, step, step, step," and "Exhale, step, step, step," as you start to warm up.

Move in rhythm: Start to pick up your pace, so that your arms get involved. Find a comfortable rhythm, one in which you can match your movement with your breath. For example, "Inhale, step, step, step, step," and "Exhale, step, step, step, step." Swing your arms or even raise them above your head from time to time in rhythm with your breath.

Challenge yourself: Set the interval timer using the Verge Mobile App, or just glance at your watch. Pick up your pace for one minute. Push it a bit. You want your heart pumping. A good way to know if you're working hard enough is to try singing "Old McDonald Had a Farm." If you can sing it easily, then you need to work harder. After a minute or so, slow down your pace to recover for thirty seconds. Then do it again. You can set your interval timer to different settings (sixty/thirty, forty/twenty). You can also ball-park your intervals with the second hand on your watch. It keeps you honest and makes you work harder.

Cool down: As you get within a few minutes from your home or car, slow down your pace. Scan your body and notice sensations. Are your muscles speaking to you? How do your feet feel when touching the ground? Notice your lower back and your shoulders. What do you feel there? Check out your surroundings, the sky and the landscape. Check in with what it feels like to see life in high definition. Notice the energy surge throughout your systems. Allow yourself to drink it all in.

Rest: When you're finished with your walk, sit down or, even better, lie down. Please do not skip this step; it's very important. The final rest is where you get to really experience your natural state, and, more often than not, it's worth its weight in gold. Close your eyes. Notice the subtle sensations arising in your body. Notice the silence in your mind. Feel the high-voltage energy pulsing through you. Enjoy this moment of silence and stillness and allow yourself to bask in the experience of being fully alive.

Practice Support

Moving your body settles your mind and your nervous system in a different way than any other practice. You know that a good butt-kicking, sweat-drenched hike or spin class can wring you out from the inside. Use the template to transform your exercise routine into an opportunity to settle your busy mind and feel awake and fully alive. In this practice you directly experience your natural state — especially your bright body.

Stay Consistent

The best advice I can give you is to move your body every day —
even if it's simply a fifteen-minute walk. Make time to do a little
something every day. Every practice, whether it's short and easy
or super-challenging, will be worthwhile. And don't blow yourself out of the water by going too hard too fast. Remember, start
small, stay steady, and build from there.

The Right Attitudes

This may sound obvious, but if you don't enjoy moving your
body, you're not going to do it. My suggestion is to change your
attitude toward movement and find something that you enjoy.
Then stop calling it exercise. Here are some attitudes that may
help.

Keep it light: Being too serious about exercising takes the joy
out of movement. If you can keep your sense of humor about the
whole thing, you may find yourself going longer and harder.

Don't judge: Your body feels different from day to day. Some
days you may rock and roll, and other days you may only crawl.
Acknowledge your highs and lows, but commit to doing something. This is how you build a consistent practice. Judging yourself harshly just adds to your drama and drains your energy.

Let go of what's not working: I used to snowboard, but I don't
anymore. I found that it wasn't as enjoyable for me as skiing. Stop
wasting your time doing activities that don't make you feel empowered and energized. If the body-pump class you used to love
doesn't feel good for your body anymore, then stop going! Move
the way your body wants to move. If you slow down enough to
listen, your body will tell you loud and clear what's working and
what's not. It may all change next week anyway.

Remember the view: When you're having trouble finding the
motivation to put on your running shoes after work, try doing the

Primer Practice Remember the View. Pause for a few moments and close your eyes. Remember how great you felt after your last run. Really remember how your body felt, how your mind felt clear, and how relaxed you felt. Remembering the view may be all you need to get yourself out the door.

Be kind: Nike has been telling us for decades to "Just do it." I might add, "But be nice about it." You don't have to beat yourself up to get moving every day. Actually, the more you shower yourself with kindness, the more you will enjoy moving. Cultivate a kind, patient inner dialogue, the kind a supportive coach would use to talk to a first grader. Maintaining a gentle "You got this" attitude can change your relationship to moving your body. Also, be grateful for what you're able to do and let go of what you're not — bum knees and all!

> Remembering the view may be all you need to get yourself out the door.

When you move with the intention of synchronizing mind and body, you release tension from places you didn't even realize were tight. Synchronizing your mind and body is really powerful. It has a distinct way of smoothing out your energy by steadying your systems. It works at the cellular level to turn on your lights and brighten your mood. It burns through the mental junk that's no longer necessary to hold in your mind.

Synchronizing your mind and body using the practice template is a game changer. It turns your workouts and everyday physical activities into a vehicle for shifting beyond busyness and directly experiencing the space in which you feel awake and fully alive from your head to your toes.

CHAPTER TEN

Meet My Mind

At a Glance: Verge Practice #3

Purpose   *Meet My Mind* is a beginner meditation practice in which you become familiar with how your mind works by synchronizing your mind and body in stillness and silence. During practice you not only notice your busy mind, but also occasionally shift beyond it and experience the space of your naturally clear mind.

Benefits   Synchronizing your mind and body in stillness and silence gives you increased focus, sharper perceptions and senses, reduced chronic tension and stress, increased joy and cheerfulness, and an enhanced sense of well-being.

How-To   After prepping your space and taking your seat, you'll close your eyes and follow these guidelines:

1. Place your attention on your breath.
2. Notice if you become distracted from observing your breath.
3. Be kind. Don't judge.
4. Place your attention back on your breath. Repeat.

Online and on the Verge Mobile App: *Meditation Instruction; Focused Deep Breathing 10-Minute Practice; Focused Deep Breathing 20-Minute Practice; Meet My Mind Practice Timer.*

My busy mind ruled my life for far too long. Yanked around by doubt, fear, expectation, comparison, and judgment, I've said stupid things, acted and reacted unconsciously, put others on pedestals, and at times put myself above others.

My fascination with human potential and my appreciation for space, stillness, and silence led me to meditation. Over the years I've spent hundreds of hours in silence, staring at the contents of my mind. I've since become somewhat of a cheerleader for this ancient and powerfully transformative practice. I enthusiastically teach both moving and seated meditation and will talk to anyone willing to listen about the long-term benefits of this life-changing practice.

I'll spare you the cheers and the pom-poms and give it to you straight up. If you really want to show up and shine, if you want to really suck the marrow out of each moment, you'll want to really take a close look at how your mind operates. If you want to be awake for this precious moment of life, one you can't do over, you'll want to understand what the heck your busy mind is so busy doing.

After staring at it long enough, you start to see what's not running smoothly, what's jammed, and what needs to be cleared away.

The purpose of this Verge Practice is to get to know how your mind works. Meeting your mind is like investigating your car engine. After staring at it long enough, you start to see what's not running smoothly, what's jammed, and what needs to be cleared away. By staring straight at your thoughts, you become acquainted with your mental engine, so to speak.

Meet My Mind is a beginner mindfulness meditation practice during which you synchronize your mind and body in stillness and silence. You do this by focusing on your breath as a way not only to settle your mind, but also to connect to your body. Synchronizing like this is a way to bring your mental activity into balance with your heart rate and nervous system. It's a way to drop below the level of mental noise into a more physical or fuller direct sensory experience.

Meet My Mind is done by simply sitting still and noticing. You notice if you are:

- Distracted or right here right now
- Not aware or aware
- Busy or clear
- Asleep or awake
- Shut down or engaged
- Dull or alert
- Active or passive

> It's a way to drop below the level of mental noise into a more physical or fuller direct sensory experience.

I could go on and on. When you sit still and just notice, you become familiar with your repetitive thoughts, destructive thoughts, brilliant thoughts, and everything in between. You get to know what it feels like to be awake and alive in the moment.

Verge Practice: *Meet My Mind*

The toolbox of *Notice This Moment* practices prepares you to sit still and notice for longer periods of time. Although *Notice This Moment* practices are done anywhere and at any time, your meditation practice is done when you've planned a specific period of time to sit down and be still.

This Verge Practice, this mindful meditation, is the next step of your mental strength training. Meditation is a way of becoming familiar with your mind by sitting still, getting quiet, and noticing. You're not trying to stop your thoughts or empty your mind. You're simply sitting and noticing. In sitting still and focusing on your breath, you recognize when you're distracted and become *aware* when you are *not aware*. You've already done this in other practices. Now you're just going to do it for a longer period of time.

Meditation is a fully experiential practice, one in which you learn *as* you practice. In other words, you can't learn to meditate by just reading a book. You have to practice. I offer you just a few instructions below, and I'll continue to support you during the guided meditations found on the Verge Mobile App. Do your best to listen to the guided practices every day. Mornings are the best time for most. I've provided you with a couple of different durations to choose from.

> You can't learn to meditate by just reading a book. You have to practice.

Prep Your Space

You already have everything you need to meditate. You don't need a meditation room in your house to meet your mind. You don't even need a room! You can meditate in your car, on a park bench, even in your office. It's best, however, to clear whatever space you're in of unnecessary clutter and distraction. Clean surroundings will help you settle down. You don't have to go overboard, just do your best and then don't worry about a little clutter or an old couch. There's no perfect place to meditate. Why? Because your mind is always with you and there is no place, no matter where, that is without distraction.

Next, turn off the ringer on your phone and computer. Ask your family members to leave you alone. Send your pets away. Even though it may seem cozy to have your dog or cat on your lap while you meditate, trust me, it will be a distraction. Close the windows if there's too much noise outside. Since you'll rely on guided meditations in the beginning, set up your device to play. Eventually you'll practice on your own, and in that case you'll want to set a timer.

Take Your Seat

Find a comfortable seat. It can be on your couch with both feet on the floor, at your desk, or on a cushion. Sit in an upright but relaxed position. In other words, don't be too rigid, but don't slouch either. If you get too comfy, you're likely to fall asleep. Your spine should be erect but at ease. Place your hands palms down on your thighs. Oh, and you don't have to sit cross-legged — ever.

Meditation Practice: Focused Deep Breathing

Meet My Mind is a beginner meditation practice. The instructions are simple, so don't try to complicate them. Keep it simple, and you will have an easier time staying consistent. Also, there's no "perfect" when it comes to meditation, and you can't be "bad" at meditating. You either practice it, or you don't. After prepping your space and taking your seat, you'll close your eyes and follow these guidelines:

1. Place your attention on your breath.
2. Notice if you become distracted from observing your breath.
3. Be kind. Don't judge.
4. Place your attention back on your breath. Repeat.

> There's no "perfect" when it comes to meditation, and you can't be "bad" at meditating. You either practice it, or you don't.

1. Place Your Attention on Your Breath

Once you're seated and ready for practice, place your attention on your breath, your natural breath, and settle in for a few moments.

Then begin to notice how your breath feels in the area below your navel, your lower belly. Don't change your breathing; just notice the subtle lifting and lowering of your lower belly as you breathe. Focusing on the breath is the most common way to start a meditation session. Your breath is always accessible and easy to find. Paying attention to the sound and the physical sensations of breathing for a few minutes starts the process of synchronizing your mind and body. It's calming and settling and prepares you to meet your mind.

After a few minutes of paying attention to your natural breath, you'll shift into a more specific way of breathing called Focused Deep Breathing. This way of breathing works for many people when they are learning to meditate. It helps shift the location of your attention; it no longer resides solely in your mind but extends to the rest of your body as well.

You're going to breathe at a ratio of one to two, so that it takes you twice as long to exhale as to inhale. Extending your exhalation so that it's longer than your inhalation has a way of settling your mind and nervous system. It holds your attention perhaps even more than the breathing pace of the Counting Breath practice and is useful when practicing for longer durations.

For this breathing practice you can use two counts for the inhale and four counts for the exhale, three and six, or four and eight. We'll try this using three and six, but if that ratio doesn't work for you, you can change it. The point isn't to hyperventilate or pass out. You want the ratio to feel comfortable, so that you stay with it. The counting helps you stay focused.

As you do this, you'll continue to hold your attention on counting your breath while also noticing your body. Notice how your chest and belly expand during your inhalation and deflate during your extended exhalation.

1. Breathe in slowly while counting to three.
2. Pause for a count of one.

3. Breathe out slowly while counting to six.
4. Pause for a count of one.
5. Once again, "Inhale, two, three, pause; exhale, two, three, four, five, six, pause."
6. Continue to breathe this way for the entire practice or until your guided meditation says to relax your breath.

2. Notice If You Become Distracted from Observing Your Breath

As you pay attention to your breath, you may notice your thoughts are still firing nonstop. It's okay. You're going to think during meditation. Your mind will continue to generate thoughts. It's what minds do. Your mind is made for thinking. Meeting your mind is not about stopping your thoughts; it's about noticing them. So when you notice yourself thinking, don't freak out or get disappointed. Just notice and move to Step 3.

3. Be Kind, Don't Judge

You're not going to stop your mind from thinking, so you might as well stop judging yourself every time you have a thought. A key ingredient to sticking with a meditation practice is to be kind and patient. You *will* get distracted. The great news is that when you become aware that you're distracted, it's a sign that your practice is working. Remember, this mindfulness meditation is about becoming familiar with your mind and all the busy stuff that goes on in there. Recognizing distraction is the mental strength training, remember? Noticing is like doing a bicep curl. Instead of judging yourself when you notice your busy mind, celebrate. Seriously, when you notice you're distracted, give yourself a mental high five, put your hand on your heart, or simply smile.

The great news is that when you become aware that you're distracted, it's a sign that your practice is working.

4. Place Your Attention Back on Your Breath

After noticing you've become distracted, then giving yourself some love or a mental high five, your final step is to direct your mind back to your next breath. Come back to Focused Deep Breathing and counting in the ratio of one to two. Repeat. Repeat. Repeat.

Postpractice Pause

When your timer goes off or the guided practice finishes, take a moment to acknowledge how you're feeling, just as you did after moving your body. Are you calmer or more stable? Does your body feel relaxed or less tense? Maybe you don't feel calmer or more relaxed. Maybe you feel more frazzled, because your mind felt busy during your practice. That's okay too. Some days you'll feel busier than others. Some days you may fall asleep in your practice. Remember, there's no perfect meditation practice, and you cannot be bad at doing it. So after your practice, thank yourself for showing up and meeting your mind. Acknowledge any shift of perspective or insight you may have experienced, and then go on with your day. Good job.

Benefits of *Meet My Mind*

Meditation can change the neural pathways of your brain, so that you are more focused and less reactive and, yes, have less chronic stress. The scientific research on the benefits of meditation goes wide and deep. The benefits are outstanding and compelling. Surf the internet for some of the research findings, and you may feel compelled to run out to buy your very own meditation cushion. Seriously, though, here are a few benefits consistent meditation practice can offer:

The benefits are outstanding and compelling.

- Increased focus
- Sharper perceptions and senses
- Deeper trust in your natural intelligence
- Reduced chronic tension and stress
- Reduced blood pressure
- Reduced anxiety
- Increased joy and cheerfulness
- Less struggle and edginess
- An enhanced sense of well-being

Practice Support

Meet My Mind is an introduction to what I hope will be a lifelong practice. As my meditation teachers, Scott and Nancy McBride, often say, meditation is different from anything you've ever done before. It's different, because instead of being pulled around by your busy mind, you're shifting your perspective by looking directly at your busy mind. The only way to really understand meditation is to practice it, and establishing a consistent meditation practice takes curiosity and commitment.

I suggest using the guided meditation practices on the Verge Mobile App right away. Listen to them every day for a few weeks and then seek out more support. Although there are many online programs and podcasts to choose from, studies show that beginning meditation students who participate in a group series are more likely to stick with a daily practice longer. Find a beginner program taught by a reputable meditation teacher. Guided practices are designed to get you started, but in order to dive deeper you'll want to get into a live class setting.

Staying Consistent

There are no benefits to practicing meditation once in a while. It's like going to the gym once a month and expecting your body to change. Your brain changes from consistent practice. It's simple science. Being consistent is essential. Here are some tips that can help.

Start small, stay steady, and build from there: Short sessions every day are much more effective for being consistent than longer sessions once a week. Start small with my guided practices. Stay steady by practicing every day. Build from there by trying longer practices and by seeking out teachers in your area.

Practice at the same time every day: Most people find early morning or late evening to be the optimal time to consistently practice. It doesn't matter when you practice, as long as you practice. If you need to skip your regular morning practice, don't sweat it. Find another time during the day to get at least a short practice in.

Use guided meditations: Don't suffer through your own practice when starting out. Use the tools available. It's okay to listen to the same guided practice over and over for a month straight if it helps you to stay consistent.

Understand the instructions: Since your breath is always there to pay attention to, it's easy to take for granted or overlook. Understanding the steps of the practice and the various breathing exercises you can choose from helps to create a container for your practice. The instructions frame your practice.

The Right Attitudes

Keep it light: Remember, take your practice seriously, but don't take yourself so seriously in your practice. Be willing to laugh at your busy mind and the crazy ways you distract yourself. If your practice isn't somewhat light and joyful, you will simply not continue it for long.

Stop trying: Remember, you cannot force yourself to stop thinking. It just won't work! Thoughts will continue to come and go. Instead, try giving yourself permission to let go and enjoy the wild ride of meeting your mind.

Drop all expectations: Every practice is going to be different. This you can count on. In other words, don't expect to be clear and calm during every practice, especially at first.

Be kind: It's incredibly important to shower yourself with love, patience, and kindness during your meditation practice. *Be Kind* is one of the Verge Strategies you'll learn more about in Part IV. Being kind will not only make your practice smoother and more enjoyable, it will also carry over into your daily life. We can all use more kindness and love. Start with yourself in your meditation practice, and let it grow. If you notice yourself getting impatient, use one of the following tips:

Say "There, there, sweetheart": I learned an easy and effective practice from my meditation teacher Scott McBride. I use it during my practice as a reminder to be patient with myself. If your mind is particularly busy, put your right hand on your heart and say, "There, there, sweetheart." It's simple kindness that goes straight to the heart. If this phrase doesn't work, use another term of endearment that speaks to you.

Use a gentle gesture: If you notice you've been swept away into distraction, treat yourself as you would have wanted to be treated when you were a small child and you made a silly mistake or fell down and scraped your knee. When you fly away on a wild journey to some fantasy vacation, put your hand on your heart, shoulder, or cheek, and smile. A gentle gesture can shift you right back to this moment without stirring up negative stuff.

Online and on the Verge Mobile App

The practice I offer you is only one way of meeting your mind. There are different ways to meditate. I've included a Body Scan meditation and a practice on connecting to your senses on the

Verge Mobile App for you to play with. Test them out and mix up your practices from day to day. You're just stepping up to the starting line of what I hope will be a long, beautiful journey of slowing down, showing up, and meeting your mind. Check out the Online Support page for a full list of what I'm offering.

Ending at the Beginning

I wrote and rewrote this chapter several times. I struggled with how to condense this enormous topic into just a few pages. I finally decided to keep it very simple by offering you a beginner meditation practice — a simple way to settle down and meet your mind.

Although the instructions are straightforward, the benefits can be life changing. By synchronizing your mind and body in stillness and silence, you not only notice your busy mind, but also shift beyond it and experience the space of your naturally clear mind. Be willing to look under the hood and get to know how you operate. This is only the beginning of what I hope will become a lifelong practice for you.

CHAPTER ELEVEN

Notes to Self

At a Glance: Verge Practice #4

Purpose *Notes to Self* is a practice through which you become aware of your inner dialogue and adopt a more honest and inspiring way to relate to yourself. It's also a way to interrupt your busy mind and your habitual mental patterns with reminders, questions, and intentions.

Benefits This practice will help you consistently redirect your thoughts and energy and enable you to shift into a more confident and compassionate way of living.

How-To *Notes to Self* reframes your actions and words. When you become more aware of your inner dialogue, you'll find ways to turn negative self-talk into gentle coaching or genuine motivational talk. You will use:

- *Reminders:* Direct statements to help you snap out of a daze and wake up in this moment
- *Questions:* Inquiries to direct your focus, actions, and words
- *Intentions:* Empowering words to help you direct your energy and bring purpose to what you're doing

Online and on the Verge Mobile App: You can sign up to receive *Notes to Self* notifications on the Verge Mobile App. You'll also find a list of suggested *Notes to Self* on my website, www.carabradley.net.

Years ago, I found myself struggling and straining in an intense hip-opening pose accurately named the Frog, when all of a sudden I realized that I was forcing my body into a place I had no business being in. In a flash, I saw the insanity. What the hell was I doing? I recognized that this was not a onetime kind of forcing. In that glimpse of clarity, I woke up and knew I'd been forcing myself into not only the Frog pose but also other situations in my life.

I heard myself ask, "What if you didn't force it? What if you let go and gave yourself permission to rest instead? What would that feel like?" With each gentle question I asked, I seemed to let go of a little bit of tension. A sense of ease began to emerge, like the sweet summer air after a thunderstorm. From somewhere deep inside, I seemed to be whispering, "Stop trying so hard." Something shifted during that pose. A tight fist inside of me began to release. I had a gut feeling my realization about forcing wasn't purely about the Frog pose.

From that point forward, I practiced yoga in an entirely new way. Instead of throwing myself into some pretzel shape, I listened to my body and how it seemed to want to move. This slight shift of perspective turned my practice upside down. Instead of forcing my body into poses, I turned my mind away from the need to get somewhere special and became curious about what I experienced. I became familiar with moments of strain and struggle and moments of ease and peace.

At first I had to remind myself to stop forcing, so I adopted a handful of questions to ask myself throughout my practice, questions like, "Can I rest in this moment?" and "Can I be at ease right now?" I also repeated gentle phrases to remind myself to pay attention to how I was moving, reminders like, "Allow," "Be kind," and "Let it go." Shifting my inner dialogue with questions and phrases seemed to work. I noticed I was relaxing more during my yoga practice and eventually began to relax more often everywhere else.

How I talked to myself was changing how I moved in the world. Honest questions and direct reminders helped me make friends with myself. My inner dialogue helped me align my actions with how I wanted to live. My words ignited and reignited my desire to be fully alive.

> My inner dialogue helped me align my actions with how I wanted to live.

Verge Practice: *Notes to Self*

"Remind," "ask," and "intend" are three ways to chat with yourself, three ways to align your actions with how you want to live. *Notes to Self* is a practice in coaching yourself to show up and be available to experience this moment fully. Elements of this practice are sometimes gentle and sometimes not-so-gentle reminders, questions, and intentions to wake up, show up, and shine.

Your reminders, questions, and intentions are meant to stop you in your tracks and redirect your attention and your energy. They're meant to interrupt you in the middle of what you're doing or thinking and make you pause to notice if you're stuck on autopilot or caught in your busy mind. By shifting your inner dialogue from negative, muddled, or chatty to positive and empowering, you direct your attention to what matters most to you and to how you want to experience your life. Your *Notes to Self* will shift your perspective from muted or frazzled to vivid and bright. Remind, ask, and intend — three ways of chatting with yourself — are three ways to wake up and show up on purpose.

You talk to yourself all the time anyway. This practice simply makes you aware of the words you're using and offers you a powerful way to continue to direct your attention. You'll adopt words and phrases that will help settle you down or pump you up. I'll help you collect and create your personal *Notes to Self*, words that energize you and can snap you out of destructive behavior or negative self-talk. The reminders, questions, and intentions can shift you into a more confident and compassionate way of chatting with yourself and inspire you to show up and experience your life directly.

Let's get started.

Reminders

Reminders are *messages that help you notice where you are, what you're doing, and where you want to go.* Think of them as a heads-up or a tap on the back. Reminders can be tender or bold. They are phrases that direct you to pause and listen or encourage you to change your actions or words. Reminders serve to wake you up from the trance of your busy mind. They'll shake you and stir you when you've gone into autopilot mode. Reminders will show you when you're shut down and encourage you to show up and experience the moment. Check out some of my favorite reminders:

> Reminders serve to wake you up from the trance of your busy mind.

- Stay calm.
- Be available for those around you.
- Embrace everything.
- Find a way.
- You've got this.

- Forcing doesn't work.
- This moment is enough.
- Practice patience.
- Be kind.
- Be helpful.
- Being overwhelmed is not an option.
- Celebrate life.

Questions

Leading questions can *direct your focus, actions, and words*. You'll ask a question, but not worry about the response. Asking sincere questions is enough to elicit an answer — and the answer may not come through in words. Oftentimes your answers arrive as subtle sensations. Sometimes you may suddenly smile, laugh, or even cry.

For example, when I'm struggling in a seated meditation practice, I'll ask myself, "Can you let go of resistance?" Sometimes I'll repeat it four or five times. I often relax just by asking the question. I feel my shoulders drop and my mind perk up. Asking the question often elicits the answer.

Asking the question is what's important for this practice. The point is to interrupt your habitual mental patterns such as worrying, doubting, or judging. Ask the question and you'll stop yourself in your tracks long enough to redirect your attention. Do this often enough, and you'll weaken the mental patterns that no longer support you. Here are some of my favorite questions:

- Does this make me feel bright?
- Can I meet this moment?
- What is real for me right now?
- Am I distracted or right here right now?
- Am I showing up or shutting down?
- Can I drop this drama?

- How can I feel fully alive right now?
- What is most important to me right now?
- Am I struggling with what is happening?
- Can I be kind to all those around me?
- Am I trying to control?
- Can I be at ease?
- Can I allow everything to be just as it is?

Intentions

Intentions, when set with clarity and conviction, are hugely powerful. They're a *commitment to carry out an action or behavior* and provide *a framework to set your priorities.*

Like reminders and questions, intentions will interrupt you from your busy mind. They will make you pause and notice your thoughts or actions. While reminders are more direct statements to snap you out of a daze, intentions are more like invitations to shift your attention.

I begin my intentions by saying "May I." Here are a few of my favorites.

May I:

- Be at ease.
- Have peace.
- Allow others to be free.
- Be bold.
- Drop my need to control.
- Be fearless.
- Be honest.
- Be real.
- Be kind
- Let go.
- Be positive.
- Let go of expectations.

- Allow everything to be as it is.
- Kick ass (had to include this one just to keep it real).

Getting Started

This Verge Practice helps you stay accountable to how you're living. It will help you interrupt negative thoughts that drain your energy, so that you can refocus your attention on what really matters. In many ways, this practice turns you into your own life coach.

Notes to Self takes no extra time, but does require a willingness to be honest about how you talk to yourself. You also have to be willing to pull together your own set of reminders, questions, and intentions. At first you may feel awkward talking to yourself in this way, but over time it will become second nature and kind of fun. In fact, this practice may not only change the way you speak to yourself, but also how you speak to others.

> *Notes to Self* takes no extra time, but does require a willingness to be honest about how you talk to yourself.

◆ GUT CHECK:
   CHOOSING YOUR *NOTES TO SELF*

In the exercise below, you're going to write out two reminders, two questions, and two intentions. These are your starters for *Notes to Self* for the next few weeks. Feel free to use my suggestions. Don't worry, you can change these and adopt new ones anytime. Nothing is set in stone. You'll want to be in a quiet frame of mind, so pause and take a few deep breaths before writing. Use your journal or the space below:

My reminders:

1. _____

2. _____

My questions:

1. _____

2. _____

My intentions:

1. _____

2. _____

Practice Support

It's important to remember that there's no right or wrong way to do this practice. Start small and keep it simple. Adopt some of my suggestions to begin with, and then create your own. Don't take on too many too fast, because you'll likely burn out and drop the practice before you ever enjoy any of the benefits. Here's my advice for setting up your practice and sticking with it.

Consistency

Be consistent: At first you may not believe that reminders, questions, and intentions can work for you. That's why it's important to commit to a few and to say them routinely, right from the beginning. Start by saying a reminder or intention or asking a question before breakfast, lunch, and dinner. Pause for a breath or two. Done.

Use technology: Your devices could be the best way to remember to practice. Copy your reminders, questions, and intentions onto your phone, tablets, and computer — somewhere, anywhere you'll see them. Set up a gong or a chime to gently ring and display one of your notes. The Verge Mobile App can do this for you.

Use sticky notes: Write out your notes on brightly colored sticky notes and paste them everywhere — in your car, on your monitor, or on your refrigerator. As you learned earlier, a great note for your steering wheel is "No speed, no struggle."

Use bells and thresholds: Find any sort of noise or transition that occurs consistently as a way to remind you to practice. Red lights, getting in and out of your car, brushing your teeth — all are regular occurrences.

The Right Attitudes

Keep it light: This is a must-have attitude when getting started. Make your reminders fun. You should smile when your gentle gong goes off on your phone reminding you to "Be fully alive" or that "You've got this." When your reminders are fun, you're more likely to put them into action.

Keep it real and be original: This practice has to feel right, not gooey or sappy, if you know what I mean. It's about shifting your perspective from busy to clear, dull to bright, and shut down to open. It has to feel genuine, or you'll drop this practice like a hot potato. If my suggestions don't work for you, don't use them. Notice what fits and what needs to be tweaked. Make up your own stuff, and keep it real for you.

Be flexible: Your notes will change daily depending on your mood, the weather, and your schedule. Give yourself permission to mix things up, and your practice will stay fresh. Some days I wake up and set an intention to "Live fearlessly," while other days I simply put my hand on my heart and remind myself to "Be kind and patient." Base your practice on what is relevant in the moment, and your inner dialogue will support you in many ways.

Be playful: I love this instruction. This practice should be joy-filled and fun! Don't be so serious. I have a hokey reminder: "Experience the incredible lightness of being!" This can shock me out of one of my intense moods and help me to smile and relax.

Be bold: Why not? What do you have to lose? I love bold intentions, such as the quote by St. Ignatius that one of my daughters taped above the window in her dorm room; it reads, "Go forth and set the world on fire."

Online and on the Verge Mobile App

Sign up to receive *Notes to Self* notifications on the Verge Mobile App. You can adjust the settings to receive only those reminders, questions, or intentions that speak to you at the time of day you think would most inspire you. You'll also find a list of suggested *Notes to Self* on my website.

Notes to Self may seem cumbersome at first, especially if you set yourself up with notes and buzzers on your phone. Do what you can to stick with it; otherwise you'll forget to practice. The rings, boings, and chirps will support you as you get started. You're sort of like a newborn doe getting used to her long, skinny legs. You'll need to lean on this support until you're up and running.

I used to have twenty or so *Notes to Self* on my phone every day. Over time, I've silenced most of them. "Be fearless" rings at 9:00 AM, "Show up fully" rings at noon, and "Celebrate life" rings at 5:00 PM. The others ring weekly on different days of the week. I continue to ask myself questions during my yoga and meditation practices and as I move through my daily activities.

When your reminders, questions, and intentions are genuine, you'll feel the charge. They'll provide you with a spark of clarity or quick hit of high-voltage energy. Sprinkling your *Notes to Self* throughout your life is well worth a little effort. Why not set yourself up for success? Why not coach yourself to feel as empowered and energized as you possibly can? Why not do everything you can to live your life fully? Why not?

PART IV

VERGE
STRATEGIES

CHAPTER TWELVE

Be in Sync

At a Glance: Verge Strategy #1

Purpose   *Be in Sync* is a simple strategy to help you maintain clarity and balance in your life. It's a way of tuning in to your mind and body to tell if they're synchronized, aligned, and working together.

Benefits   Being in sync is your direct experience of this moment from a clear mind, bright body, and open heart. When you're in sync, you feel any or all of the following: vibrant, energized, empowered, ready, aligned, at ease, happy, peaceful, relaxed, available, steady, and confident.

How-To   Follow these steps:

1. Ask, "Am I in sync or out of sync?"
2. Pause and give yourself a moment to assess your state.
3. If you find that you are in sync and feeling good, then keep on doing what you're doing!
4. If you are out of sync, use *silence*, *stillness*, or *rhythm* to stabilize and synchronize your mind and body.

Sitting on my deck on an early summer morning is about as close to heaven as it gets. The fresh air and sweet sounds of the birds bring me joy. As I sip my coffee and gaze up at the sky, I am at peace. Absorbed in the moment, I feel connected to my surroundings; I feel awake and alive. During those sweet moments I'm carried beyond my worries to a place of being in harmony with life. These early mornings on my deck remind me how nature always finds balance. I learned to trust that I can find balance too.

The Verge Strategies are easy-to-remember ways to help you stay clear and stable. They are quick check-ins with your mind, body, and heart to make sure that you're balanced. The Verge Strategies aren't something you do just once a day like taking vitamins. Think about them more like checking the time. You check the time on your watch, and in an instant you know if you're going to be early or late. Verge Strategies are ways to notice if you're stuck in your busy mind.

You have your own strategies for healthy living, for how to stay well rested and well fed. The Verge Strategies are a set of questions to help you stay awake and aware. The Verge Strategies enable you to show up in this moment and live on the verge.

Verge Strategy: *Be in Sync*

The first Verge Strategy, *Be in Sync*, is a way of tuning in to your mind and body to tell if they're synchronized, aligned, and working together. You check in with your state throughout your day just as you would check the time on your watch. Instead of barreling through life with a busy mind, you pause periodically and tune in to your mind and body.

Ask yourself throughout your day, "Am I in sync or out of sync?"

Asking this question *is* the strategy. Doing so makes you pause long enough to notice your state of being. You're not looking for a detailed answer. You'll sense the answer in the same breath that you ask the question. It will seem to emerge from deep inside your body. You just know when you're in sync or out of sync. It's like riding a bike — you know when you're off balance and you know how to rebalance yourself. More often than not, you'll find that you're out of sync. (If you were in sync, you wouldn't be called to ask the question in the first place.)

In sync or out of sync? Let's take a closer look at what this means.

Being out of Sync

If you are stuck in your busy mind, your mind and body are out of sync. When you are distracted and drained, your experience is muted and your senses are dulled. You are not experiencing the moment in high definition. You are living from your busy mind and feel disconnected from the sensations arising in your body.

When you're out of sync, you feel any or all of the following: unsettled, unstable, ungrounded, irritable, tired, hurried, stressed, impatient, judgmental, and anxious. I'm sure you could add another couple of dozen words to this list. You feel off balance if something is really weighing on your mind. You feel unstable if you're feeling like a victim in a relationship. You feel out of sorts when you have a head cold. You get the point.

Being in Sync

Being in sync is your direct experience of this moment from a clear mind, bright body, and open heart. It is when you tune in to your full sensory experience. You feel awake and fully alive. You feel energized and empowered, steady and stable.

Being in sync is your natural state. When you're in sync, you feel any or all of the following: vibrant, energized, empowered, ready, aligned, at ease, happy, peaceful, relaxed, available, steady, and confident. Being in sync goes beyond words. It's a sense of being whole. It's a feeling of being in harmony and alignment in both your inner and outer worlds. You can be in sync anytime — while on a run, lying on the beach and listening to the ocean, spinning at a spin class, floating in a pool, working on a jigsaw puzzle, or hiking in the woods. You can be in sync when gardening, chopping carrots, playing music or chess, or making love.

Being in sync is your natural state.

This Verge Strategy is simple. Ask the question. Pause for the response. Start checking in with yourself all the time — when you wake up, in the shower, in the car, before a meeting, standing in line, during your workout, having drinks with friends.

If you find that you are in sync and feeling good, then keep on doing what you're doing! When you know you are out of sync, you want to get steady and stable as quickly as possible.

Although my deck is a perfect environment for me to feel balanced and in harmony, I can't always run back to my deck to synchronize my mind and body. The most effective way I've found to steady and stabilize my mind and body is to spend a few moments in *silence, stillness,* or *rhythm.*

Finding Time in Silence

I've grown to appreciate that silence truly is golden. It settles and steadies me in a matter of minutes. I didn't always feel this way. I used to surround myself with noise. I'd fall asleep with the television blaring, have music playing in my car and home, and talk, talk, talk until my throat was sore. Now I seek silence every day.

There are two types of noise and two types of silence — outer and inner. It's important to understand the difference.

Outer Noise

Outer noise is the stuff you hear in your environment: talking, music, machines humming. Are you aware that there's noise almost everywhere you go these days? Music plays in stores, restaurants, and hotel lobbies. Beeps, gongs, and whistles sound all around us. News is broadcast 24/7. Our species is overstimulated with outer noise. We are conditioned to require constant music and entertainment. It's become the norm.

Inner Noise

Inner noise is the phenomenon of being in a quiet room yet feeling as though a whole crowd of people are talking to you all at once. It's the voices in your head continually reminding you to do this or to figure out that. Inner noise is your busy mind in action, continuously bouncing around from one thought to the next and filling your mind with constant chatter.

Outer Silence

You can stop the incessant outer noise by finding pockets of outer silence. Turn off the noisemakers such as your laptop or television. Your mind and nervous system will naturally settle down. Your car is a great place to find outer silence — this means turning off the news, music, and your phone. Drive in silence, and you turn your car into a four-wheeled Zen center. Take a few minutes of peace and quiet. Take control of outer-noise pollution in your car, office, and home, and you'll notice a shift in your energy right away.

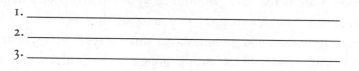

GUT CHECK:
OUTER SILENCE IN YOUR LIFE

Off the top of your head, list three areas in your life where you already have outer silence (for example, when running without music, cooking, in your office, or gardening). If you have a hard time coming up with three areas, then note areas where you *could* choose to have outer silence in your life:

1. _____

2. _____

3. _____

Inner Silence

Inner silence *cannot* be found by shutting down your computer or by being alone in your bedroom. Inner silence emerges from the space beyond your busy mind. You can't force it to emerge or make it stay. Inner silence arises from your natural state — when your mind is calm. It's a sense of being quiet from the inside out, when your mind is steady and your body is relaxed. You can learn to access inner silence through practice.

The Primer Practices are effective ways to quiet your inner noise and glimpse inner silence. These short practices shift you beyond your busy mind for a few moments, giving you a glimpse of your natural state. The Verge Practices *Move My Body* and *Meet My Mind* help to calm, steady, and stabilize your mind and body for a longer period of time. These powerful practices reveal your inner world, generally a busy inner world that over time will settle down and relax.

At first, there's anything but inner silence during your practices, and you might feel as though you're hanging out at Grand Central Station. Eventually, you catch glimpses of the space in between thoughts, moments that may feel like the most silent silence and the most spacious space you've ever experienced. Synchronizing mind and body and accessing inner silence are inextricably linked; they cultivate and reinforce each other.

Inner silence leaves an indelible mark. It feels like coming home. It feels so good to be steady and stable. It feels so good to be energized and in harmony. It feels like home to be in sync. Once you get to know inner silence, you'll want nothing else but to live in that space all the time.

Finding Time in Stillness

Years ago, when my family and I were in Italy, my then four-year-old daughter, Julianna, looked out the hotel window from the fourth floor one afternoon and said, "Mommy, there's a dead man in the chair down there!" When I looked out, I saw a man napping in a small yard behind a restaurant. She was witnessing the afternoon siesta — that delicious pause that is still somewhat a part of Italian culture. As they say in Italy, *Che dolce far niente*, which means, "How sweet it is to do nothing." While the Italian restaurateur was living *la bella vita*, my American daughter, unaccustomed to seeing someone resting in the middle of the day, saw a dead man. Busyness starts early in our culture.

Like outer and inner noise and silence, there are outer and inner busyness and stillness.

Outer Busyness

Most people really do believe that "getting more done" will lead to more happiness. We boast about being "crazy busy" and criticize ourselves for lingering or pausing. Where does stillness fit into our busy lives?

We're trained to be productive from an early age. Nowadays, children have learned how to "pack it in" by kindergarten. By the time they're in middle school, they're bound to their colorful assignment books stocked with lists, due dates, and homework. My kids used to march in the door after school and start right at it, diligently crossing off assignments. "Like little soldiers," I used to think, until I started enforcing play and rest time before homework. Outer busyness is cultural, and it occupies most of our waking day.

Inner Busyness

Inner busyness, like inner noise, is the stuff that occupies your busy mind. It's not always a bad place to be; it's actually where great stuff happens, like problem solving and planning. It's just that there's little stillness or silence there. There's no time to recharge. The machine is always running. If you get stuck in inner busyness, you'll feel like the hamster on the wheel going around and around with no end in sight.

For me inner busyness feels like having too many documents and images open on my computer. There are so many windows on the screen that I can't find my desktop. It also slows down the entire system. Nothing seems to work efficiently. Multitasking is sort of the same. You're thinking about multiple things to do at the same time and can't find the space to think clearly.

Outer Stillness

Stop moving and you'll experience outer stillness. Pause, right now, without fixing your shirt or shifting in your chair. When you step off the raceway and give yourself permission to stop moving, you will feel yourself settle in a matter of moments. The few minutes of rest at the end of your workout or yoga class are great examples of outer stillness and how readily available it is. Let's face it, you have five minutes to be still.

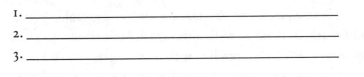

◆   GUT CHECK:
    OUTER STILLNESS IN YOUR LIFE

List three areas where you experience inner or outer stillness (for example, meditating in the morning or watching the sunset). Again, if you can't think of times during your day when you're able to be still, jot down a few options to experiment with (such as pausing in your car before heading into your office, or taking a five-minute rest after eating lunch):

1. _____

2. _____

3. _____

Inner Stillness

Like inner silence, inner stillness is not something you can manufacture or try to achieve. It's a quality of being that cannot be explained, but must instead be experienced. When you shift beyond your busy mind, you slip into a space where time seems to stand still. If you hang out there long enough, you'll sense yourself become still.

You access inner stillness by stabilizing your mind and body. The various Primer Practices you learned can shift you into this space. Being in sync and experiencing inner stillness are interwoven. One doesn't exist without the other. To meet your life from this inner stillness is a great relief. Like inner silence, inner stillness feels like coming home. It's where you feel awake and fully alive.

Finding Time in Rhythm

Rhythm, a steady beat, a repeated pattern of movement or sound, is found everywhere, from the beating of your heart to the dripping of water from the faucet. Your body relaxes and stabilizes when in rhythm. We synchronize with the beating drum, the breath of our partner sleeping beside us, or the cadence of our running partner. Start to become aware of the rhythms inside of you and all around you. The four primal rhythms humans experience most often are:

Heartbeat
Breathing
Walking
Rocking

These elements of rhythm are always available. You could add music in there as well, although it isn't always available or appropriate. The bottom line is that as long as you're breathing, you have the opportunity to synchronize your mind and body.

The Primer Practices, especially Box Breathing, utilize rhythmic breathing to stabilize and balance your mind and body. Try one of the Primer Practices next time you're feeling anxious or stressed. It's easy to do and very effective.

 GUT CHECK:
FEEL YOUR RHYTHM

List three areas in your life where you notice rhythm. For example, I get into a great rhythm when I hike, and I feel the rhythm of my breath when I rake leaves. If you've never thought about the rhythms naturally occurring in your life, then think of something you do consistently every day that can be done rhythmically (for example, walking from your car to your place of work or wiping down your kitchen countertop):

1. _____
2. _____
3. _____

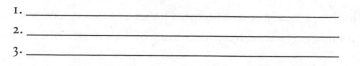

Be in Sync is a simple strategy to maintain stability and balance in your life. Instead of barreling through life, pushing and exhausting yourself in each activity, you instead tune in and take care of yourself. By asking, "Am I in sync or out of sync?" you pause and give yourself a moment to assess your state. Asking the question elicits the response. In a matter of one or two breaths you'll know if you're in sync or out of sync, and you'll know what you need to be steady and stable. In inner silence, inner stillness, and the primal rhythms of your heartbeat, breath, and body, you synchronize and shift from thinking to feeling and from doing to being. Being in sync, in body and mind, is a great relief. It feels like coming home to your natural state of clear mind, bright body, and open heart. It feels like being awake and fully alive.

Am I in sync or out of sync?

CHAPTER THIRTEEN

Be Kind

At a Glance: Verge Strategy #2

Purpose   *Be Kind* is a strategy of checking in on habitual self-judgment and feelings of unworthiness and interrupting negative self-talk with words of encouragement and kindness. This strategy is how you make friends with yourself.

Benefits   Remembering to be kind opens your heart and helps you to be more available to yourself and others. It allows you to recognize the goodness in others and yourself. By making friends with yourself, you learn to consistently shift beyond negative self-talk and access the space where you are clear, bright, and open.

How-To   *Be Kind* is a practical strategy. It starts with invoking kindness, tenderness, and a bit of humor in your life. You do this by:

1. Tuning in to your experience.
2. Noticing your inner dialogue.
3. Interrupting unkind or mean dialogue with a kind word, a tender gesture, or some comic relief, including:

    Offering yourself the same sort of delightful encouragement you might give your love object.

    Placing your hand on your heart and saying, "There, there, sweetheart," "You got this," or "Don't sweat it."

    Repeating the *Be Kind* reminders:

May I feel safe.	May I be happy.
May I have peace.	May I be at ease.

used to be a typical type A personality. Some may claim I still am. I've certainly done my fair share of striving and pushing. I've also spent years judging myself: my body, my leadership style, and my ability to compose a coherent sentence. You name it, and I've judged it. I'm as normal as it gets when it comes to good ol' American-style beating myself up and throwing myself under the bus. So when I was first introduced to the Buddhist practice of loving-kindness, that is, making friends with myself, I did what most people do — I resisted. I translated being kind to myself as being soft, and type A's don't do soft.

Making friends with myself felt like trying to move tectonic plates. I faced deeply rooted patterns that didn't want to budge. But when they did, even a degree or two, there was big-time transformation. When I found the courage to be kind to myself, I started to relax. I learned to embrace myself, and others, with compassion, tenderness, and even humor.

> When you notice yourself being less than nice to yourself, you're going to offer yourself a small gesture of kindness, humor, or tenderness.

As I made friends with myself, I actually started to — gulp — love myself. It happened slowly, and over time I began to see all the ways I'd been hiding from myself. Being kind shifted me beyond all my self-inflicted drama and opened me up to exploring my life, where I felt really excited to just be me — with my former type A–ness and all.

Verge Strategy: *Be Kind*

Be Kind is a strategy of checking in on habitual self-judgment and feelings of unworthiness. When you notice yourself being less than nice to yourself, you're going to offer yourself a small gesture of kindness, humor, or tenderness. Once you start noticing your tendencies to judge, be impatient, and even be cruel to yourself, you'll recognize that kindness, tenderness, and even a little bit of humor are what make the world go 'round. *Be Kind* is a strategy that'll just rock your world as it did mine.

I often jokingly tell my friends that being a yoga teacher is sometimes a little like being a priest. When I run into Verge students in stores and restaurants in the Main Line suburbs of Philadelphia, I hear confessions like, "I haven't been to Verge in three months," "I'm just not good at yoga," or "I tried meditation, but I really can't sit still." Having been raised going to Catholic Confession, I'll often joke with them by saying, "No problem. Just do three Up Dogs and three Down Dogs, and you're good!"

And so it goes. "I'm not good enough" and "I'm too distracted." "I can't do a handstand" and "I can't sit still." "She's so flexible" and "I'm so fat." Over and over, day in and day out, for our entire lives.

Feeling unworthy is taking you on the long road to nowhere. Judging and comparing yourself to others is a royal waste of time. Beating yourself up for not working out, for eating the pint of mocha fudge ice cream in the freezer, or for quitting early during meditation practice is useless. Feeling like crap about yourself does nothing to make you feel alive and everything to make you feel more like crap. Unless you stop

> Feeling like crap about yourself does nothing to make you feel alive and everything to make you feel more like crap.

judging yourself and start making friends with yourself, you'll keep spinning your wheels on the proverbial road to nowhere.

Basic Friendliness

Loving-kindness, called *metta* in Pali, is not a romantic type of love, but rather a behavior, an offering of friendliness toward all living beings — including yourself. Especially yourself. And if that's not a tall enough order, *metta* is a kind of *unconditional* loving-kindness, which means you need to completely embrace yourself — the good, the bad, and the seemingly ugly.

We were born with an innate capacity to love unconditionally, and most of us are in constant search of ways to share our joy. We also share a deep longing to be loved unconditionally and to connect with others. Life situations, however, often get in the way, and our genuine longing to love and be loved gets warped all out of proportion or shoved down deep below protective patterns, societal conditioning, life experiences, and even incessant busyness.

Be kind to yourself as you are right now.

You already know how to love. You're already friendly. You're already patient and kind. You don't need to try to do anything to be better. Be kind to yourself as you are right now. That's the strategy.

Choose Your Love Object!

An easy way to start making friends with yourself is to consider how you interact with a toddler or, even better, your dog or cat. Animals bring out the best in people; they bring out our natural friendliness and they don't talk back to us. Hang out with a warm fuzzy friend for a few minutes, and you'll shift from rigid to gooey.

Young children and animals provide you with uncomplicated

relationships. Notice how you feel a warm, cozy glow when you're with them. Not all relationships have this effect. That warm, cozy glow doesn't surface with everyone we hang out with. For this reason, we'll call your pet or child — or anything else you connect with from a place of unconditional love — your "love object." Yep, you read it correctly — your love object. Stay with me here.

Next time you're with your dog, cat, baby, or friend's baby, notice how you speak, the words you use and the tone of your voice. Watch your playfulness and gentleness. I find it so easy to be authentically joyful and loving with my rescue dog, Joey. He's my love object of choice, and when I'm with him, I feel light and kind. Joey, my little mix of dachshund and terrier, has, in many ways, taught me how to love myself.

By highlighting pets and babies, I'm not saying your older children cannot be your love objects, but at some point your relationship with your children becomes more complicated. I can attest to this, having two daughters in their early twenties. Their inevitable need for independence, their desire to do things "their way," has added to the dynamics of our quality family time. Our relationships with our children become more complicated as they age, so why not keep it simple? Stick with pets or babies.

Next time you're with your love object, notice your lightheartedness and joy. Notice what it feels like in your body. Notice the words you use. Notice how a sense of compassion and joy seems to emerge from your heart and fill you to the brim. This is the warm, cozy glow of being kind and loving.

You can turn the direction of this warm, cozy glow around and aim it directly at yourself. You can turn yourself into a love object. Can you talk to yourself the way you talk to your dog?

Think about it the next time you're ready to slam yourself with harsh judgment. Would you speak like that to your cute little pup? Checking in and offering yourself some love and kindness in a gentle, even joyful way is how you make friends with yourself; it's the strategy *Be Kind*.

How to Be Kind

Be Kind is a practical strategy. It starts with invoking kindness, tenderness, and a bit of humor in your life, not just once in a while but all the time. As with the Verge Strategy *Be in Sync*, you tune in to your experience. For this strategy you tune in and notice your inner dialogue. If the dialogue is unkind or downright mean, you interrupt it with a kind word, a tender gesture, or some comic relief. Let's dive in.

Kindness

The definition of kindness is being friendly, generous, and considerate. Simple, right? Of course it is. You're kind to the person checking out the groceries, your neighbors, kids, and your partner. But are you kind to yourself?

Do you offer yourself a friendly high five when you finish a project at work? Do you praise yourself when you tack on an extra mile to your walk? Are you compassionate toward yourself when you're fighting a head cold?

Kindness lives within you. It arises when you get out of your own way and shift beyond your stories and supposed failures. Kindness arises when you show up in this moment and allow yourself and everything else to be just as it is.

Simple gestures can help you remember to be kind. I already mentioned one I learned from my teacher Scott McBride. When you feel stuck in a situation or a negative thought, put your right hand on your heart and say, "There, there, sweetheart." If these words aren't in your lexicon, try saying something like, "You got this," or "Don't sweat it." If these phrases don't work for you, then make something else up. What feels gentle and kind for you? Notice the words you use with your love object. How do you console your child or your dog?

Almost immediately you may feel yourself relax and your shoulders drop. It's as if you're saying to yourself, "It's okay. I know you're trying your hardest." I know this may be challenging or uncomfortable and actually feel forced at first, but I bet you'll catch on quickly. Just keep doing it. "There, there, sweetheart."

◆ GUT CHECK:
CHOOSE YOUR PHRASE

Off the top of your head, what words of kindness work for you? Write them here or in your journal. You can even record them and use them as your ring tone (I'm not joking!):

You are loved you are enough.

Humor

We can all use a little more laughter, wouldn't you say? There's nothing that lightens and brightens a tense moment like some gentle humor. You can learn to rediscover playfulness and humor in your life just by shifting the way you speak to yourself. A genuine sense of humor is another way of saying, "Lighten up." Why not reignite your playful, childlike qualities, which have been dormant in your life for perhaps decades? When did we all get so serious anyway?

My childhood nickname was Mimi. I've readopted this name when using this strategy and use it often when speaking to myself. For example, I may say out loud, "You got this, Mimi," as a way to stay light and playful. There's a kind quality about calling my-self Mimi that can stop me in the middle of a negative rant or pull me out of the dungeon of unworthiness.

 GUT CHECK:
HOW DO YOU LIGHTEN UP?

Off the top of your head, what do you do to lighten up? Do you have a funny voice, gesture, or name that makes you smile or relax? Write it here or in your journal. Why not paste it on your laptop screen?

john

make a face. think of mulaney.

Tenderness

Tenderness arises when you let life touch you deep down at your center where you're willing to open up to life as it is right now. Being tender is a way of letting down your guard and opening up to directly experience life in this moment. It may seem so ob-vious, but it wasn't to me for a long time. I often asked why I needed to "practice" being tender. The answer was simple and clear: because I had closed myself down to really being vulnerable to others and myself.

Now I usually cry at least once every day. It's not the bad kind of crying, but the good kind — a gentle expression of joy and grati-tude. I'm so often touched by the incredible beauty and goodness in the world that I'm brought to tears. Oftentimes just noticing kind-ness in others or their sincere desire to do their best can shift my tear ducts into overdrive. Being kind helps me allow my life to unfold gently, in a way that makes me available to see, taste, touch, and smell the radiant beauty of life as it is, with no filters.

Look out at the world with openness and tenderness, and

you let the world touch your soft spot, right in the center of your heart. As you open more and more, you recognize that others around you, either those close to you or those just passing you on the street, are likely struggling to be tender too.

Knowing that most people are not tender or kind to themselves has a way of piercing my heart. You may start to feel the same way. There is so much to go around. We have so much love to offer one another, but first we need to offer it to ourselves.

Be Kind Reminders

At first you're going to need to remember to be kind to yourself, especially if you're out of practice. There are a few reminders that can really help. Carry them close to you and pull them out to recite throughout the day. These reminders will interrupt your busy mind when you notice you're headed down a potentially destructive path, such as when you feel unworthy, judge or compare, or simply feel down in the dumps. These traditional reminders are used in Buddhist loving-kindness practices. Apply them to everything you do. Say them in the morning and at the end of the day. Say them during your Verge Practices. Repeat. Repeat. Repeat!

May I feel safe.
May I have peace.
May I be happy.
May I be at ease.

May I feel safe.
May I have peace.
May I be happy.
May I be at ease.

Slowly repeat the phrases to yourself either out loud or in your mind. You can say them all or pull out just one. Pause for a moment afterward, and then go about your day.

I use the phrase, "May I be at ease," throughout my day. I say it to myself when moments get tense, when doubt arises, when I am running late. I say it over and over, sometimes changing up the words: "May I rest in this moment," "May I embrace what's happening," and so on. As you learned in the Verge Practice *Notes to Self*, you can set your phrases up as reminders on your phone.

If saying these reminders feels forced at first, start by saying them to your love object. Sending your dog, cat, or baby love in this way can help you get comfortable with these powerful reminders. You can also direct these reminders to those you work with, drive by, or meet in a store. Share the love all over town, and you'll soon become more comfortable sharing it with yourself. Check in with the Verge Mobile App for a guided loving-kindness practice.

When done as a more formal loving-kindness practice, you would include other people, such as loved ones, acquaintances, and all living beings when reciting these reminders. When the practice becomes all-inclusive like this, it begins to really stir you from the inside out, awakening your capacity to love more deeply.

Being kind to myself has opened my heart in a good way, a really good way. It's helped me experience the goodness in myself and to recognize the goodness in others. I'm confident it can help you do the same. By making friends with yourself, you shift beyond distraction and drama; you slip into the space where you are clear, bright, and open. You show up in this moment and are available to shine in the world. Be kind to yourself in every way possible, and you'll live on the verge every day.

CHAPTER FOURTEEN

Let It Go, Let It Be

At a Glance: Verge Strategy #3

Purpose When you allow everything to be just as it is and let go of your need to force, fix, or flee, you become available to experience exactly what is happening in this moment. By letting go, you become liberated from the heavy burden of thinking you have to fix everything and make everyone happy.

Benefits *Let It Go, Let It Be* makes you less reactive, allowing you to have a deeper connection with others, to be more honest and easier to be around, and ultimately to have more energy and feel more awake and alive.

How-To This strategy is your invitation to investigate how you hold back and how to let go. More a way of living than a technique, it will help you, first, get to know your tendencies to force, fix, or flee and, second, build the confidence to embrace the moment instead of resisting it. You do this by:

1. Checking in with your body.
2. Asking if you are forcing, fixing, or fleeing.
3. Reminding yourself to let it go and let it be.
4. Noticing the space in your mind and body.

I'm a small business owner, so my daily life gets chaotic and sometimes messy. Conversations happen on the fly, emails are exchanged in a matter of seconds, and stuff needs to get done. It's easy to get distracted and be short with others. A few years ago, two students and an employee confronted me within a matter of two days. I had pissed off each one of these people for different reasons at different times, and they all had called me on my questionable behavior within forty-eight hours.

The details aren't important, and in the end everything was resolved. As I listened to those I'd hurt, it was difficult for me to breathe. One after another, I faced my actions. It became clear that how I was treating others was not aligned with what I was teaching. In the process of attempting to manage and grow a busy yoga business, I tried to force and fix everything and everyone along the way. In my effort to make Verge Yoga shine, I'd become a controlling and demanding person.

I'd not only exhausted myself trying to make my students happy and make my business run smoothly, but at times I'd also hurt and offended others. I knew I had to change. I'm grateful to those three people who held a mirror to my face, making me pause and look at myself. After sitting with what had transpired in those forty-eight hours, I opened my fists and turned my palms to the sky. I felt myself surrender as I said out loud, "Let go."

Verge Strategy: *Let It Go, Let It Be*

Let It Go, Let It Be is a Verge Strategy to investigate what's holding you back from doing exactly that, letting go. It's a tall order, no doubt. This is a transformative way to live. Once you understand and start to sense the freedom that letting go offers, you'll try it all the time. This strategy will accomplish two things. First, it will help you get to know your tendencies to force, fix, and flee, and, second, it will help you build the confidence to embrace the moment instead of resisting it.

Contrary to popular opinion, letting go doesn't mean being lazy or passive. It doesn't mean to dissociate or let the world pass you by. Letting go means saying yes to what's happening right now by allowing the moment to unfold without your having to control or manipulate it. Letting go is relinquishing your need to change people and situations to fit your plans. It's a strategy to live "in the flow" instead of resisting it. By embracing and facing each moment instead of forcing or avoiding it, you shift from shutting down to showing up and from being controlling to being open and available.

You can let go anywhere and at any time. First you check in with your body and notice if you're trying to force, fix, or flee. You ask yourself, "Am I trying to force (or fix or flee) this moment?" Then you'll remind yourself to let it go and let it be. You say, "Let it go, let it be." In the process of saying this you'll shift and relax. You'll experience a space in which you can let go of resistance and allow the moment to unfold naturally.

Let's go deeper.

> Letting go means saying yes to what's happening right now by allowing the moment to unfold without your having to control or manipulate it.

Check In with Your Body

Your body is a messenger. It communicates through the language of sensation. Sensations will tell you exactly what's coming up. Sensations travel at lightning speed through your nervous system. They're like alarms that go off when you're headed into a potentially charged situation, alerting you long before your busy mind gets around to realizing something's going on.

Check in with your body often, and you'll get to know the sensations associated with your tendencies to force, fix, or flee. Take a look at some of the sensations you might find familiar.

SNAPSHOT:
SENSATIONS OF FORCING, FIXING, OR FLEEING

Stomach churns or flutters	Eyes squint	Cheeks burn
Body stiffens	Throat closes	Chest swells or rises
Breath shortens	Face tightens	
	Heart pounds	

If you pay close attention, you'll get to know your body's signals right before you try to control a situation. I've learned, often the hard way, that your body offers you invaluable information and can save you from a lot of drama in the future.

Ask If You Are Forcing, Fixing, or Fleeing

Check in with yourself often enough, and you'll notice that you habitually try to control or push away situations and people when you want whatever is happening to be different than it is. The need to have life play by your rules is a surefire way to create struggle and suffering in your life. This need commonly emerges for the following reasons:

You *hold on to* what you like or what makes you feel good.

You *push away* what you don't like or what makes you feel bad.

You *ignore* what you don't want to deal with or what appears boring.

It's really very simple. You suffer when you resist what's happening right now. You suffer when you try to make what's happening different. You suffer when you force, fix, or flee. So if you check in with your body and notice even the slightest hint of stiffness, stirring, or burning, pause right away and take a breath. Before reacting ask yourself, "Right now, am I going to try to force, fix, or flee? Can I let go and meet this moment?"

Asking the questions interrupts your busy mind and destructive habits. Asking stops you in your tracks and helps you to shift into your natural state, where you're much more likely to allow than to control. In the space beyond your tendency to control you access your naturally clear mind and open heart.

So what does it mean to force, fix, or flee? The definitions are different for everyone. Let's take a look.

Right now, am I going to try to force, fix, or flee? Can I let go and meet this moment?

Forcing

Forcing is your tendency to manipulate people and situations in order to make outcomes shift in your favor. Forcing happens when you try to make something happen or try to make someone do something you want. It's what you do when you contort your body into a yoga pose before your body's ready to do it safely, or you ask your young son to practice piano after he's continually told you he really doesn't like playing the piano. We all force to some degree. It's helpful to get to know your tendencies.

Fixing

Fixing is your tendency to try to make situations better or make people behave so that you are not uncomfortable or inconvenienced. When I started becoming aware of my behavior, I realized I was a compulsive fixer. I fixed my children's issues, my problems at work, even other people's problems at work. I was a fixer of life. This didn't necessarily make me feel good. I recognized there is little space and little joy in always fixing life. At some point I realized I was going to have to stop fixing myself and start being myself. In the end, people need to make mistakes, walls need to crumble, and we all need to relax more and allow life to unfold without the help of our overly involved sticky fingers.

Are you a fixer? If so, get to know what you habitually try to fix.

Fleeing

Fleeing is your tendency to avoid or ignore uncomfortable and unpleasant situations or people. We're hard-wired to run from danger and potential threat. In the absence of real danger, this instinct goes to work to help us avoid or ignore stuff we don't want to deal with because it's unpleasant or boring. Because our brains cannot recognize the difference between real fear and perceived fear, our systems go into action, ready to fight or flee as soon as we perceive the possibility of being uncomfortable. And so it goes. We flee relationships when they become inconvenient, drop classes when they get too difficult, and skip parties if we don't want to deal with someone else who's going to be there.

What about you? Do you ignore or run away from situations or people?

Let It Go, Let It Be is your invitation to fess up and face yourself by recognizing how you deal with uncomfortable moments and unfamiliar or inconvenient situations and then interrupting your tendency to force, fix, or flee.

◆ GUT CHECK:
　　YOUR TENDENCIES TO FORCE, FIX, AND FLEE

Take a moment and write down two ways each that you force, fix, or flee. Start with the small stuff. Here are a few of my tendencies as examples. I used to try to force my daughters to clean up their bathroom (gave up on that one years ago). Sometimes I remake the bed after my husband makes it (yep, it's true). I look for a snack when faced with a challenging paragraph to write (been snacking a lot lately). What are yours?

Ways I force:

1. _____

2. _____

Ways I fix:

1. _____

2. _____

Ways I flee:

1. _____

2. _____

Reminders for *Let It Go, Let It Be*

After you've checked in with your body and asked if you were forcing, fixing, or fleeing, you're ready for a reminder, a prompt, something to make you pause before you do or say something you'll regret. Reminders are essential to letting go. *Let It Go, Let It Be* is a perfect reminder in itself. However, it's important to connect with the words. Create a few reminders for yourself and carry them with you at all times. Whichever reminders work for you, stamp them everywhere — on your computer screen, on your phone screen, on your refrigerator.

Letting go means to pause before forcing, fixing, or fleeing. It means staying with the uncomfortable, unfamiliar, and the inconvenient even if you don't want to. Letting go means giving up the need to control. It essentially means to say yes to this moment and allow everything to be just as it is.

Letting go means giving up the need to control.

Of course this is all easier said than done. As we know, life gets messy, loved ones may get sick, your partner may leave, and the shit may very well hit the fan. I'm not claiming to have a magic answer or to tell you that by snapping your fingers and shouting, "Let go!" you'll instantly be free. What I am offering you is an option, the possibility that you don't have to struggle and suffer if you consider that a shift in perspective could offer you a way to experience life differently. I'm suggesting that by allowing life to unfold without putting your sticky fingers in, you open yourself to experiencing freedom.

"Let it go, let it be." You can say it over and over. You can have a gesture to remind you. Whenever I feel my need to control emerge, like when my cheeks get hot or my throat contracts, I squeeze my fists really tight and take a deep breath as I release my fists and flip my palms toward the sky. This simple gesture has helped me tremendously. The fists make me pause, and the pause makes me take a deep breath. The deep breath reminds me to pay close attention to my words and actions, so that I do no harm. Opening my palms is a powerful act of letting go; it's my personal gesture to allow and embrace, to let it go and let it be. Nobody knows I do this — until now.

A few months ago I asked my Facebook friends to share what they do to remind themselves to let go. Here are a few comments I received:

- Gretchen, an Ironman finisher, shared: "It's not very Zen, but I close my eyes, and say, 'Inhale...shut up, shut up, shut up, shut up, shut up, shut up...exhale.'" It's her way of quieting her mind when she feels a strong urge to say something she may later regret.

- Tori, a Verge Yoga teacher, asks herself, "How much will this matter in five minutes? Five days? Five years?" If the answer is "Not much" or "Not at all" (and most of the time it's "not at all"), then she tells herself to move on and not waste another second on something that really isn't important.

Others shared the following:

- I put my hand on my heart and pause until the need to control passes.
- I say, "It's okay," three times really slowly.
- I cross my fingers really hard, so I don't lash out.
- I go for a walk and breathe in the fresh air before mouthing off or sending the self-righteous email.

Letting go begins with first being honest about your tendencies to force, fix, or flee. This strategy is just something you do over and over. At some point, you won't have to think about it as much. My advice is to start small, stay steady, and build from there. Instead of tackling the biggest inconveniences and the most difficult people — a financial issue, an ex-partner, or a boss — I suggest you start by letting go of your son's dirty laundry on the floor or the coworker who never makes the coffee. Starting small will help you build confidence and courage for the large-scale situations and people.

At first you may need sticky notes — everywhere. You may need to set bells and whistles to play on your devices, reminding you to let go. Transitions in your daily life work too, such as the moments before you walk into your house or your office. I'll often repeat, "Let it go, let it be," during my walk from my car to the doors of Verge Yoga. This strategy prepares me to stay clear, open, and out of my busy mind as I greet staff and students.

Strategy Support

The following are tips and tools to make this strategy a part of your daily life.

Letting go is cumulative: The great news is that the more you can let go, the better it feels to let go. Every time, and I mean every time, you let go of your need to control, you get stronger, which is why you want to do it all the time. Allow the car to merge in front of you, embrace your friend as she boasts about her children, let go of your need to always tell your assistant how to format the spreadsheet. Let people be on their own journey, and know that in so doing they'll give you more space to be on yours. Letting go is cumulative.

The more you can let go, the better it feels to let go.

Admit your tendencies to force, fix, or flee: You can practice meditation, yoga, and deep breathing exercises until you're blue in the face, but you won't understand what it's like to really let go until you're willing to face yourself and your habits. You need to look at your tendencies to force, fix, or flee to get to know yourself in a way you haven't in the past. I can't promise it'll be pretty, but from experience I know it'll be worth it. When you allow everything to be and let go of your need to control, you open up to experience life fully, and you're liberated from the heavy burden of thinking you have to fix everything and make everyone happy.

Light, Bright, and Liberated

A wonderfully light sense of joy arises in the space beyond forcing, fixing, or fleeing. In giving yourself permission to let go, you become kinder and more compassionate not only toward others, but also toward yourself. You open to possibilities. You immediately feel lighter and brighter. Holding on to the need to control people and situations is a heavy burden. When I decided to let go five years ago, I committed to relinquishing my need to control everything and to allowing my life to unfold more gracefully. I proclaimed a big *yes* to embracing situations and allowing others the freedom to be as they are, and over the years I've felt a huge weight lift from my shoulders. This sense of freedom has been an incredible relief.

When you let go and let be enough, an interesting thing starts to happen. You feel your shoulders relax and your heart open up. A sense of lightness and freedom comes over you like a fresh breeze sweeping past your face. When this sense of freedom bubbles up, acknowledge and appreciate it. It's exactly where you show up and shine.

CHAPTER FIFTEEN

Be Aware

At a Glance: Verge Strategy #4

Purpose   *Be Aware* helps you recognize when you're engaged and fully aware by waking up to when you're not aware. In noticing when you're unaware, you immediately become aware.

Benefits   When you're aware that you're aware, you glimpse your direct experience in this moment. This is living on the verge — your full participation in this moment when you feel awake and fully alive.

How-To   As in the other Verge Strategies, you check in with your mind and body and ask a question. For this strategy you'll ask, "Am I aware or not aware?" You'll likely find yourself at one of the five levels of awareness:

1. Busy Mind: You are *not aware* that you are *not aware*.
2. Waking Up: You are *aware* that you are *not aware*.
3. Power Pause: You are *aware* of the power in pausing.
4. Glimpsing Your Natural State: You are *aware* that you are *aware*.
5. Living on the Verge: You are *fully aware*.

How you experience this moment is very much like looking through a camera lens. You can look at the world in panorama or zoom in for a close-up. The lens can be focused, showing sharp lines, or unfocused, so that shapes are foggy and blurry. What you see depends on whether your lens is in focus, what type of filter you're using, and what type of lens you're using (telephoto, wide angle, or standard).

When you're upset or pissed off, your experience may be filtered so it feels dull or distorted. If you're trying to multitask, your experience may feel fragmented. When you are engaged and fully aware, you experience the world in high definition. Your lens is focused and crystal clear. How you experience what you're feeling and what's happening around you comes down to whether you are awake and aware or busy and asleep.

Awareness is your perception of this moment. It's how you experience life right now. When you're unaware and trapped in busy mind, life appears unfocused and sort of foggy.

Being unaware is like trying to take a picture but being unable to focus the lens. On the other hand, when you're fully aware, your perception is crystal clear. You experience life in high definition. You're aware of ideas, perceptions, and physical sensations as they arise. Being fully aware is like seeing life through a camera lens that's clear and focused.

> Awareness is your perception of this moment. It's how you experience life right now.

Verge Strategy: *Be Aware*

Be Aware is the final Verge Strategy. It helps you feel more awake and alive by recognizing when you're not aware. As in the other Verge Strategies, you check in with your mind and body and ask a question. For this strategy you'll ask, "Am I aware or not aware?" As in the other strategies, the question elicits the response. What you'll discover is that you were hanging out at one of the following five levels of awareness. Let's take a deeper look.

The Five Levels of Awareness

The five levels of awareness help you distinguish when you're aware and engaged and when you're not aware or distracted. They are like mile markers or reference points to help you determine your location, or state of mind, in any given moment. Understanding the five levels will help you to uncover where you're spending most of your time and energy. You may be surprised at what you find. The five levels of awareness are:

They are like mile markers or reference points to help you determine your location, or state of mind, in any given moment.

1. Busy Mind
2. Waking Up
3. Power Pause
4. Glimpsing Your Natural State
5. Living on the Verge

At Level 1, you're stuck in your Busy Mind, preoccupied with doing, consumed by your overflowing lists and overcrowded schedule. You can feel mentally frazzled, emotionally exhausted, and physically tense. At Level 1, you may not recognize there's a healthier and more empowering way to live. You are *not aware* that you are *not aware*.

At Level 2, Waking Up, you shift beyond busy mind and momentarily wake up out of the dream state of thinking. Your busy mind gets interrupted and you catch yourself in the middle of an angry or anxious moment or fantasizing about where you want to vacation next year. In other words, you catch yourself entrenched in drama and distraction. You are *aware* that you are *not aware*.

At Level 3, Power Pause, you experience the space beyond your busy mind long enough to pause and interrupt your habitual tendencies to worry, doubt, fear, or judge. During the pause you recognize that you can choose to either show up and be engaged or slip back into dullness, distraction, or drama. You are *aware* of the power in pausing.

At Level 4, Glimpsing Your Natural State, you shift into the space beyond your busy mind and glimpse your natural state of clear mind, bright body, and open heart. You feel stable and clear for a few moments. Although it may be short-lived, you recognize your natural state and what it feels like to be fully alive. You are *aware* that you are *aware*.

Level 5 is Living on the Verge, a metaphor for being awake. You experience life through the unfiltered lens of your natural state. You feel clear, bright, and open. You show up and shine. You are *fully aware*.

Exploring the Levels of Awareness

You float in and out of awareness all day long. Some moments you're asleep, and other moments you're awake. The five levels of awareness are simply reference points to get a handle on where you are at any given moment. There are no hard and fast descriptions of what these reference points feel like. In other words, stay flexible and experiment with them.

For example, this morning while answering emails, I noticed my eagerness to get back to editing this chapter. I was *aware* that I was *not aware*, and I also recognized that to get back to the chapter, I needed to pay attention to the emails. I paused and realized I

could remain distracted and ineffective, or I could choose to focus
and get the job done. Since I didn't want to waste time being distracted, I perked up and blasted through my responses. In those
moments, I danced in between Level 2, Waking Up,
and Level 3, Power Pause.

You do the same — you dance in and out
of awareness, on and off the verge all day
long. *Be Aware* is a strategy to help you notice where you are — aware or not aware —
and to help you spend less time and energy in
your busy mind and more time glimpsing your
natural state and living on the verge.

> You dance
> in and out of awareness,
> on and off the verge
> all day long.

Level 1: Busy Mind

You are *not aware* that you are *not aware*.

At this point, we've established we're busy people living in
busy minds. We've explored how much our culture reveres multitasking, and we overthink and overdo. We've explored how we
identify with our busy minds and have been conditioned to operate in an ocean of endless noise and information. Let's agree that
from busy mind you are simply *not aware* that you are *not aware*.

Here's a sampling of what getting stuck in busy mind might
look like:

Forgetting an appointment
Losing your cell phone — again
Zoning out in front of the TV
Finding yourself on social media — again
Eating the doughnut before realizing what you were
    doing
Arriving in your driveway not really remembering how
    you got home

You'll determine if you're stuck at Level 1 or if you're shining at Level 5 based upon what you're directly experiencing in your body, mind, and heart. Here's a summary.

Body: When your mind is frazzled, your body is too. Mental overload leads to physical tension. Depending on how you hold tension, your neck and shoulders may feel chronically sore and stiff or you may suffer from lower back pain. Studies show that when your mind is in perpetual hyperdrive, you live in chronic physical stress, taxing your systems and draining your energy reserves. Signs of stress in your body include increased inflammation and blood pressure, weight gain, and feeling sluggish.

Mind: The busy mind is often compared to a monkey jumping from tree to tree, always swinging and moving. The busy mind is a crowded and often unproductive place to live. Thinking, planning, processing, and remembering can be exhausting. Jumping around from tree to tree in your busy mind can leave you feeling frazzled and fragmented. Get to know how you feel in your busy mind, and you'll learn how to shift beyond it.

Heart: Living in a constant state of mental movement can also feel like riding a roller coaster for a few hours (or a few years). If you're easily swayed by outer opinions and circumstances, you can roll from high to low and back again all day long. Remember, drama drains your energy. Worry, doubt, and negativity trigger the stress response and can leave you feeling depleted and disconnected.

Level 2: Waking Up

You are *aware* that you are *not aware.*

The moment you notice you're distracted, you become engaged. The noticing is enough. In the exact moment you recognize your busy mind, you shift beyond it. You wake up from the trance or the dream state of overthinking and overdoing and experience the moment directly.

Waking up is recognizing the difference between being in your busy mind and being here right now. It may happen for a moment or a minute. Waking up feels like taking in a breath of fresh air or a cool breeze that suddenly blows through the window and brushes your cheek. Waking up happens the moment you take a break in the middle of your crazy-busy life and catch yourself being unaware. In that moment you experience the sweet relief from the crowding and clutter of busy mind.

Examples of waking up can include:

Catching yourself not paying attention while driving

Noticing that you've drifted off during a conference call

Sensing anger rise as your child resists your request to sit still

Feeling disappointment emerge when your colleague announces her promotion

Recognizing that you're frozen with fear as you step onto the soccer field

Body: Your body absorbs stuff from your mind. Your mental junk exhausts your body. As you become *aware* of when you are *not aware*, you wake up to the physical sensations associated with mental and emotional busyness. For example, you notice how you clench your jaw during the morning staff meeting or that your stomach tightens when you think about your son's struggle with schoolwork.

Mind: Level 2 is like stepping into a quiet room during a party and delighting in the silence. From this view, you look back into the party and see the chaos of chatter, music, and lights. When you slip into this space beyond outer and inner noise, even for a minute, you experience the space just beyond busyness and feel clearer and more relaxed.

Heart: At Level 2, you recognize how negative emotions grip or even paralyze you. Waking up from the dream state of the busy mind, you recognize how often you judge your body, your intellect, and your lack of money or time.

Being aware of when you are not aware can be very exhilarating.

Being aware of when you are not aware can be very exhilarating at first. Waking up, you experience yourself not as your thoughts or emotions, but instead as a clear mind, bright body, and open heart. You recognize how you've been unconsciously led around by your busy mind.

Level 3: Power Pause

You are *aware* of the power in pausing.

Level 3 is a turning point. It's when you realize you can intentionally choose how to live. At Level 3 you become *aware* of your power to choose your state. In other words, you experience being aware not just as a flash of a moment, but as a longer, more spacious encounter. In the space, you have more time to choose to stay awake or to go back to sleep.

Some examples of Level 3 are:

Noticing your hand reach for a second helping of mashed potatoes and pausing to breathe

Stopping yourself before you criticize your partner

Putting your hand on your heart as you notice negative self-talk

Reviewing the emotionally charged email you've written and deciding not to send it

Recognizing that you cannot do everything on your list today

Smiling at the inconvenience of a delayed flight instead of having a tantrum

At Level 3, you feel empowered. You know you don't have to be crazy busy and that you don't have to involve yourself in the small dramas of everyday life. Instead, you know you can choose how to show up in the world. You can choose to be aware of how you move and speak in the world.

Body: Your body is a mirror image of your mental state. At Level 3, as long as you're not in real danger, your nervous system shifts from tightness and tension into a calmer, more natural way of being lighter, brighter, and more at ease. Your body feels less frozen and more fluid.

Mind: At Level 3, you slip into your natural state for a prolonged moment. Picture a quarterback surveying the field for a few seconds before throwing the ball or running with it. The more time he has, the more he can choose with precision. At Level 3, you shift into your clear mind long enough to choose your response. Time seems to slow down, and you feel less hurried and frantic.

Heart: At Level 3, you recognize your moods in greater detail and choose your action or response with more preciseness. You feel better equipped to assess a situation and choose an appropriate response. You're more discerning and less impulsive. At Level 3, you pause long enough to skillfully choose your actions and words and potentially avoid unconscious or destructive behavior.

Level 4: Glimpsing Your Natural State

You are *aware* that you are *aware.*

Every so often you shift beyond the busyness of life and directly experience a surge of energy and aliveness. This happens when you pause to notice the warm sun on your face as it peeks between the clouds or hear the joyful noise of two children jumping on a trampoline. You glimpse your natural state and feel fully alive. In moments like these you are fully aware. It can arise as a sudden burst of joy or sadness. It can hit you like a brick, waking you up immediately, or it can emerge gently as a swell of deep peace. In either case, you glimpse your natural state of clear mind, bright body, and open heart. At Level 4, you are *aware* that you are *aware*.

Examples of glimpsing your natural state are:

A lingering feeling of peace during an extended vacation

A sense of time standing still when you find out someone you know has died

A feeling of tranquility when you watch the sun rise

A sense of awe when looking up at the stars

Active attention or fierce focus while dealing with a challenging problem

A surge of confidence during the final moments of a basketball game

Body: In the space beyond thoughts and emotions and in the absence of any threat of immediate danger, your nervous system will shift from the busy, high-stress state of "fight or flight" to the calmer, more relaxed state of "rest and digest." When you let go of mental overload, your body releases tension. At Level 4, you experience a sense of vitality and well-being and feel charged with high-voltage energy.

Mind: In the space beyond your busy mind, you experience life from a different vantage point and shift into an understanding that you are not your thoughts; you are not your busy mind. From this expanded view, you directly experience your world in high definition. You move and speak from the space of your naturally clear mind.

Heart: Being aware that you are aware is what I mean by "getting out of your own way." You've shifted beyond the level of drama and distraction, beyond the self-absorbed busy mind. At Level 4, you shift into the space that feels more "we" and less "me." Your heart is open, and you move through life with a genuine confidence and fearlessness.

Level 5: Living on the Verge

You are *fully aware*.

As a child, I luckily spent many days playing in the attic, behind the shed, and in the woods right next to a busy highway. Back in those days, my daily life sparkled like the sun on the water. The possibilities for fun and adventure were limitless.

Children's minds are naturally open and carefree. They spend their waking hours engaged in every situation, open to every possibility, living in the space where they are naturally awake and fully alive.

As a child, you were fully aware. You can yearn to return to those days, or you can lean into your life right now and experience such aliveness again. The purity of your childhood awareness is not gone. It continues to move and speak through you. You glimpse vivid moments of being awake and fully alive in your daily life. You glimpse them in your practices. If you glimpse, glimpse, glimpse often enough, you begin to trust a glimpse not as some extraordinary peak experience, but instead as a real, direct experience of your natural state. This is living on the verge — it's showing up, open and available in this moment and feeling awake and fully alive.

As a child, you were fully aware.

Direct experiences of living on the verge come in many packages and can arrive in ordinary moments. Living on the verge happens not when you're *thinking*, but when you're *being*; not when you're *doing*, but when you're *experiencing* life fully.

Examples of living on the verge are:

Being fully engaged in playing the piano
Being intensely involved in an emergency situation
Laughing until you cry
Crying until you laugh
Singing at the top of your lungs

Sprinting toward the finish line
Being absorbed in an open-air concert
Waterskiing on a calm lake
Bathing your newborn before bedtime
Sitting bedside with your ailing parent
Hugging or petting your dog or cat

When you shift to Level 5, Living on the Verge, you experience the world in high definition and with high-voltage energy. Your mind is clear, your body is bright, and your heart is wide open. You are awake and fully alive. You are fully aware of what's happening around you and inside of you.

Living on the verge, you wake up, show up, and shine.

Living on the verge happens not when you're *thinking*, but when you're *being*; not when you're *doing*, but when you're *experiencing* life fully.

PART V

SHOW UP
AND SHINE

CHAPTER SIXTEEN

Coming Home

Y ou are meant to shine — every day. It's your most natural way of being. When you clear the clutter and settle the chaos that weigh you down and hold you back, you arrive in a wide-open space where you're naturally awake. What you don't realize when living from the level of your busy mind is that every day, every moment, every conversation, and in every move you make, you are invited to wake up, show up, and shine.

Shining isn't something you learn to do; it's how you *show up to be*. You can't search for it — *you are it*. Wake up from the trance of your busy mind, and you're there, you see clearly, in high definition. Get out of your own way, drop the drama, and you're there, open, available, and ready to access high-voltage energy. Shift into the space where you're fully aware, and you feel yourself relax and let go. Show up in this exact moment — on the verge — and you're naturally radiant. You're fully alive.

Shining is a metaphor for what happens when you directly experience life with all your senses. It's the result of being 100 percent engaged in this exact moment right here and now. Shining is what happens when you live on the verge.

When you shine, you do everything better, with attentiveness and excellence. Everything you

> When you shine, you do everything better, with attentiveness and excellence.

see, taste, smell, hear, and touch is more vivid and in high definition. Your words are truthful and genuine. You're available to
others. You're charged with high-voltage energy. You radiate a
brilliant sense of peace and possibility.

Shining doesn't *always* mean breaking the record, winning
the award, or closing the deal (but sometimes it does). You have
moments every day when you shine. You shine when you show
up to really listen or say just the right words of encouragement
or acknowledgment to someone. You shine when you pause to
allow the sun to warm your face or stay attentive to your daughter
when shopping for her prom dress. You shine when you stay calm
during a heated negotiation or tell the truth even if it may not be
the popular answer.

"Shining" is a catchall term for the many different expres-
sions of what you feel when you're not preoccupied with thinking
and doing. Shining is another way to say *being*, simply *being right
here and now*. Shining is a way of moving through the world as
clear mind, bright body, and open heart.

Shining — once you glimpse it, you'll want more. Get to
know what it feels like to shine, and you'll recognize when you're
not shining. Become familiar with shining in your practices, and
you'll shine more in your life.

You shine every day, sometimes for a mere minute or two, sometimes for an hour. You'll know it
when it happens, because time seems to stand still
and everything around you seems to release and
relax. Shining feels like a huge relief — like when
the clouds part and the sun shines on your face or
when you get to put down your heavy baggage after walking through the airport. When you let go of what dulls your senses
and drains your energy, you show up and shine, and in many ways
it feels like coming home.

Get to know
what it feels like to
shine, and you'll
recognize when
you're not shining.

Give this Primer Practice a try. Get intimate with the space in which you already shine, and you will find yourself shining all the time.

 PRIMER PRACTICE:
COMING HOME

Take a moment's pause with me. This will take only one minute.

1. Set your timer for one minute.
2. Close your eyes and take a few deep breaths.
3. Place your hand on your heart.
4. Quickly scan your body.
5. Look directly at your mind and notice the space. You're not looking at thoughts or focusing on your breath. You're looking directly at the space in your mind. You can do this. Don't try; just relax. Again, look at the wide-open space of your clear mind.
6. Allow thoughts, emotions, or noises to move in and out of the space without placing importance on anything moving through your mind. Treat every thought, sound, and sensation equally.
7. Keep coming back to simply looking at the space. Don't try to grab it or hold on to it. This is the space in which you're already fully aware. Notice the relief. Notice the space. Notice your clear mind. Notice the sense of coming home.

How Do You Wake Up, Show Up, and Shine?

There are infinite ways to live on the verge, and there are countless ways to get there. One thing is for sure: you won't get there from your busy mind. In order to really wake up, show up, and shine, you'll need to shift beyond it. Once you do, there are endless ways for you to shine. I'm offering you four possibilities, four ways you can show up, shine, and live on the verge. Let's take a look.

Leaning into ripe opportunities: To really shine in your life, you'll want to explore shifting past the boundary of what's familiar into the edges of what's uncomfortable — moments I call ripe opportunities.

Trusting intelligence: Your body is like an incredibly sensitive information network that carries messages through sensations. Trust these nonverbal sensations to guide you, and you'll access your natural intelligence.

Welcoming peace: Rest in the space of your naturally clear mind, bright body, and open heart, and you'll welcome peace in every moment.

Experiencing fearlessness: Awakening the courage to face your fears head-on results in defusing and rendering those fears powerless and allows you to shine a light on anything false, untrue, or artificial.

Beyond Words, the Ocean, and the Waves

These four possibilities of living on the verge just scratch the surface. At some point, your experience of what it means to shine will go beyond your capacity to describe it. Trying to explain being fully aware to yourself or anyone else seems to lessen it's authenticity and oftentimes the profoundness of what you experienced.

The insufficiency of words to describe the simultaneous emptiness and fullness of aliveness is the very reason painters, musicians, and other artists are inspired to create. When words don't suffice, poets turn to metaphor. For millennia poets, scholars, and sages have used the nature of the ocean as a way to describe the ultimately indescribable qualities of being awake. Although my version may not be as eloquent as those of the poets who've come before me, I hope it paints a picture of how you may experience life when you wake up, show up, and shine.

Let's say you're spending the day at the beach, and you decide to go into the water to relax on your float. When you're floating on the water, you're focused on the waves, on what's happening on top of the ocean. You notice the weather and the ebb and flow of the waves. You look around at the boats, at people floating around you. It's very pleasant, and you're having a lovely time. Even though the bottom of the ocean exists beneath you, you don't think much about it. With your head above the water, you pay attention to only a small portion of the ocean. There's nothing essentially wrong with floating.

However, if all you ever do is hang out on the waves, if you never dive deeper and check out what's happening below the surface, you'll always be at the mercy of the ever-changing waves and the weather. Some days the ocean is choppy and rough, while other days it's calmer. You may encounter wind and rain or perhaps a light breeze and sun. These constantly changing elements dictate the quality of your experience.

Floating on the waves and paying attention to only the surface of the ocean are much like living from your busy mind. Whether you're stuck in drama or drifting aimlessly in distraction, your experience is easily swayed by the changing environment. Floating on the surface of ever-shifting thoughts and moods, you're easily swayed by outside influences such as a work deadline, a cranky child, or the recent gossip in the neighborhood. Whether it's rough waves or a stubborn boss, you experience life as a continuous series of ups and downs with not much to hold on to and nothing to stand on. Does this sound familiar?

There's a more peaceful and more powerful way to live.

You're back at the beach, and this time you become curious and decide to go scuba diving to check out what's happening on the ocean floor. Hanging out down there, you look around. It's different from the surface — so vast and so still. There's no noise.

You feel a tremendous sense of peace, as you're gently rocked side to side by the ocean's slow, deep rhythm.

The bottom of the ocean is like the space you experience when your mind and body are synchronized. It's the silence and stillness you feel when you're fully aware. At the bottom of the ocean your body feels fully alive, and your mind is at ease. A serene contentment washes over you. You feel a huge release as you exhale, like the "aah" at the end of a tough workout or workday.

To live on the verge, to be awake and fully alive, is to recognize that you are the waves *and* the ocean floor. You are the water and everything in the water. You are the ocean. You are its stillness and its movement. Shift beyond your busy mind into the space of your natural state, and you become the ocean noticing the waves; you become the space noticing thoughts and recognizing emotions.

Live on the verge, and you float on the waves of life while trusting that you are also part of the vast ocean beneath them. It's living in the world as the whole ocean while allowing yourself to delight in the waves at the surface.

When you know yourself as the ocean, your world — inside and out — becomes infinitely brighter. You not only glimpse the space beyond your busy mind, but you know that you *are* the space. You feel like you've come home, which is exactly where you shine.

CHAPTER SEVENTEEN

Leaning into Ripe Opportunities

"Potential." The word carries promise — a lot of promise. It's been sprinkled throughout the self-help world for decades and has been used and overused to the point that, for most people, it's lost its meaning. You'll see the word "potential" pasted everywhere from phone ads to the label on a bottle of nail polish. It appears so frequently and is used in so many different contexts, you're likely numb to its true significance.

According to *Merriam-Webster*, "potential" is defined as "a latent excellence or ability that may or may not be developed." Realizing potential is to wake up to the best of who you are already. Potential already exists. It waits in every moment for you to wake up and show up.

When you shift beyond the doubt, fear, and expectations of your busy mind, you slip into your natural state of clarity, vitality, and availability. This is where you realize potential. When you live from your busy mind, you are too preoccupied to develop your latent excellence. When you shift beyond busyness and drama, you meet the space and opportunity to realize potential. When you show up in this space, you shine.

> Realizing potential is to wake up to the best of who you are already.

Potential emerges when you say the right thing, figure out the answer just in time, or pick up the phone instead of holding back.

It's those moments when life seems to "click." Potential manifests in how you move and speak in the world. It's in the tone you use with your children, in the compassion you offer your elderly parent. It's in how well you listen during a board meeting, in how you acknowledge coworkers, and in how you greet a stranger.

Your potential shines through in seemingly small ways and big ways — all the time — like when you prepare a beautiful holiday dinner, nail your closing argument, set a goal and reach it, create or break a habit, or make a commitment to a relationship. Big or small is relative; what's more important is that you start acknowledging moments throughout your day when you step up to the plate, take the swing, and whack the ball out of the park — even if it's simply hosting a really great party.

 GUT CHECK:
HOW DO YOU SHOW UP AND SHINE?

Without thinking or hesitating, write down three areas of your life where your potential consistently shines through. And, yes, you have three. They can include actions, ways of living, or relationships (for example, playing the piano, lifting weights, coding computer programs, eating well, gardening, selling cars, caring for your children, or running a business):

1. _____
2. _____
3. _____

At first you may feel awkward acknowledging that you shine when, say, you cook an awesome breakfast, but after a while you'll recognize it all matters. Whatever you do with the qualities of attention and intention — from making breakfast to selling a house — counts as showing up and shining.

Ripe Opportunities

Although all the seemingly small moments really add up to a life well lived, there are other opportunities to realize potential, other ways that you show up and shine, ways that most people seem to speed by and miss or avoid altogether and ways that pay big dividends. I call them *ripe opportunities.*

Ripe opportunities reside in uncomfortable moments and unfamiliar situations. They happen all the time. Since you likely don't seek out ways to be uncomfortable, you may be missing ripe opportunities to realize potential every day.

Let's say you are asked to deliver a talk in front of a large crowd when you least expect it, or you ski off the chair lift and suddenly find yourself at the crest of a black-diamond run with no other way down. How do you meet moments when you're thrown out of your comfort zone or into unknown territory? Does your heart start to race just thinking about it? Do you start sweating? Do you dive into the challenge, or do you look to run away as fast as possible?

Facing an unfamiliar situation or pressing up against the boundaries of your comfort zone may make you a bit shaky. One thing is for sure: when you face moments like these, at the edge of where you're comfortable or familiar, you are on the verge.

In this exact moment between a moment ago and a moment from now you are invited to live on the verge. It doesn't matter if this exact moment is sprinkled with fairy dust or smells like skunk, you are invited just the same. In every moment you are invited to wake up, show up, and shine.

Ripe opportunities are such invitations. They invite you to lean in and get curious about what you're capable of doing and who you're capable of being. They invite you

> At the edge of where you're comfortable or familiar, you are on the verge.

to realize potential. Ripe opportunities invite you to cross the boundaries into the uncomfortable and the unknown and to show up and shine.

Ripe opportunities appear all around you all the time. They can look like a traffic jam when you're late for a meeting or a sick child on a day when you had a full day of personal plans. Ripe opportunities are those moments when you feel squeezed or stuck between a rock and a hard place. They are incredibly fruitful places to practice being awake and aware. A slow computer, a flat tire, a call from the school nurse, or losing your luggage can all be ripe opportunities. Ripe opportunities are everywhere. They are prime moments to shine. The only question is how you are showing up.

Ripe opportunities are those moments when you feel squeezed or stuck between a rock and a hard place.

 GUT CHECK:
YOUR RIPE OPPORTUNITIES

Without thinking or hesitating, write down three ripe opportunities in your life right now that you're avoiding or ignoring. Be honest. It's no use hiding any longer. (For example, you check out when your kids fight, you always have the TV on because you don't like silence, your messy roommate drives you nuts, you always give up toward the end of your spin class, or you hold back too often in meetings.)

1. _____

2. _____

3. _____

Please know this isn't about feeling bad about yourself. That's a waste of energy. Put your hand on your heart right now and smile. This Gut Check is about becoming aware of how you may be missing ripe opportunities to grow, to realize potential, and to show up and shine in your life. So no pity party here, okay? Becoming aware of ripe opportunities is where life gets very interesting. Let me explain.

Lean into Your Edges and Boundaries

To really show up and shine, it's not enough to just be calm and clear. It requires action. You need to *be in the world*. The missing ingredient for many is having the courage and confidence to lean into the edges of life.

To realize potential you not only have to show up in this moment, but you also have to stay with the moment. Artists, scientists, and athletes lean into the uncomfortable and the unknown all the time. In fact, they thrive by doing so — and with practice so will you.

Leaning in means to press into and poke around the edge of what's comfortable and familiar. Your edge is the threshold between what is known and unknown, between comfortable and uncomfortable. Athletes, business owners, and parents press up against the edge of what they think they're capable of doing every day. It's the only way to grow and evolve.

To realize potential you not only have to show up in this moment, but you also have to stay with the moment.

The issue is you're likely conditioned to either gloss over or avoid the uncomfortable and the unknown. You should know that leaning in goes against everything you want to do. Humans are conditioned to avoid what is unpleasant and uncomfortable and to seek out what is pleasant and familiar. Our natural instinct is to run from uncertainty. We hate living in the unknown and will do anything — *anything* — to avoid facing the truth that we have no idea what is going to happen next. We are genetically coded to avoid uncomfortable situations. The bottom line is that we don't want to feel uneasy about anything!

So why even try to lean in? Because it is precisely in the center of the fire where you experience life in high definition. It's there, on the edge of what is familiar and comfortable, where you feel the charge of high-voltage energy rush through you.

> It's there, on the edge of what is familiar and comfortable, where you feel the charge of high-voltage energy rush through you.

When life gets uncomfortable, most of us look for the exit doors. It seems easier to avoid than to lean in. If you want to show up and shine, you'll need to face what you avoid, ignore, or suppress and see it all as ripe opportunities. This is where your practices can support you.

Practice Leaning In

Your practices are the perfect place to safely explore leaning into your edges. They help you recognize ripe opportunities. If you're resisting your evening walk or your morning meditation, lean in and get curious. Stay with it. These are ripe opportunities.

You will experience doubt, fear, and resistance. You will try to convince yourself to skip your practice. You'll even meet edges before you even begin to practice. Watch your thoughts. Watch your emotions. Notice your body. Stay with it. Do this every time. They are all ripe opportunities for growth.

There will be times when you're practicing *Move My Body* or *Meet My Mind* when you want to run away. This is exactly the edge that you want to lean into. It's often said that understanding a yoga pose begins exactly when you want to get out of it.

How you do one thing, you do all things. What you do in your practice, you do in life. Get to your practice, and it will shed light on how and where you're stuck in life. Lean in during practice, and you'll lean into life. Show up and shine in practice, and you'll show up and shine in life.

CHAPTER EIGHTEEN

Trusting Intelligence

You are already awake. You are already fully alive. You need only listen and trust.

Beyond the static of your busy mind, you're able to sense the energy arising from your body — an intelligence that always flows through you. When you're fully aware of this intelligence, it will wake you up and remind you that you are not your doubts, your fears, or your roles and responsibilities. Shift beyond your mental noise and trust this intelligence, and you will experience a sense of aliveness that is so natural and familiar, it will feel like coming home.

The intelligence that moves through you is part of you and every living being. It has been given many names, including consciousness, *prana*, and *chi*. Call it what you will, but why not go beyond words and beliefs and investigate this intelligence yourself? Whatever expression it takes, this intelligence is already right here. You only need to listen and trust.

Beyond the Static of Everyday Busyness

Your body is communicating with you all the time. Sensations arise from your body and inform your nervous system, offering you nonverbal messages and fresh insights. Your body constantly sends you alerts and notifications. You move. You breathe. You scratch an itch. You lick your lips. You know when to sleep, eat, drink, blink your eyes, go to the bathroom. This intelligence keeps your body alive — and you already trust it.

But there's so much more to being alive than just eating, sleeping, and pooping. There's a deeper level of intelligence that you may be missing, an intelligence that shows up beyond thinking. If you tune in beyond the busyness, you sense this intelligence. It's a deeper, subtler sensation that is always ready to inform you. Without fail you'll know when you're sucked into drama or distraction, and you'll recognize when you're awake and aware. Beyond words or thinking, your body always tells you the truth. Wake up and get curious, because this intelligence is your latent excellence called "potential."

> There's a deeper level of intelligence that you may be missing.

Sensing this deep intelligence is at your fingertips. You feel it when your mind is steady. You experience it when your body is calm. Show up in this moment, where you're naturally clear and focused, and you directly experience this intelligence at full strength.

With practice you can become skilled at speaking the language of sensation. Listen carefully, for it comes and goes quickly. It informs you when to lean in. It tells you when to let go. It emerges beyond the static of your noisy life. You sense it in only one place — in the space between a moment ago and a moment from now, the space called the Verge. Listen to this deep intelligence. Live from it, and you'll know what you need and what to do in every moment and ripe opportunity. Trust the intelligence emerging from your body, and you will undoubtedly show up and shine.

Your practices give you the confidence to trust this intelligence, to trust you know what you need and what to do. Your practices build your trust in the energetic feel of your natural intelligence, and you begin to feel it all the time. Allow it to guide your life, and you'll discover that this intelligence emerges continuously in different ways, through all your senses. In other words, don't *think* about it too much. Instead, allow yourself to become familiar with a variety of subtle messages. Take a look at this Snapshot offering some of the sensations commonly experienced.

⊙ SNAPSHOT:
SUBTLE MESSAGES FROM YOUR
INTELLIGENT BODY

Uneasiness	Jumpiness	Heaviness
Agitation	Queasiness	Disturbance
Dullness	Stirring	Tightness

While finishing my edits for Part V of this book, I suddenly came down with what felt like the flu. My body ached, my neck felt stiff, and I fluctuated between having chills and feeling feverish. I sensed deep down that it wasn't the flu. I sensed it had more to do with my uneasiness about how to express what I really wanted to say in Part V.

Instead of fighting or ignoring these messages, I listened to them and trusted them to inform me of what I needed to do to get the job done. I trusted my intelligence to guide me. I spent a few extra days focused on Part V, reworking every chapter. My flu symptoms disappeared, and I went on with my writing.

Although your messages may not always seem so obvious, they are always available. Step beyond the static of your busy mind and tune in to the subtle energy shifts. At some point, you'll drop words altogether and simply trust your intelligence and the messages arising throughout your body. Ultimately it goes beyond words and beyond thinking. You can't really learn about it from a book; it must be directly experienced. You need to tune in and investigate your energy, your body, and the messages flowing through you all the time. This Primer Practice is an effective way to start connecting with this intelligence.

 PRIMER PRACTICE:
BODY SCAN

A quick inner body scan can help you settle down, so you can better detect the shifts and sensations in your body. Follow the instructions below or tune in to the Verge Mobile App for a guided Body Scan practice.

1. Lie down on the floor or a couch where you can stretch your legs out. Place your arms comfortably at your sides, palms face up.
2. Set your timer for ten minutes.
3. Close your eyes.
4. Take five deep breaths.
5. Bring your attention to your feet. Linger on your feet for a few breaths and notice everything you can about your feet. Scan each of your toes, the bottoms and tops of your feet, your heels and ankles. Do the same as you move your attention up your body to your lower legs, knees, upper legs, hips, lower back, torso, upper back and chest, arms and hands, shoulders, neck, skull, and face.
6. As you scan your body, name any sensation you notice. For example, "My feet feel cold," "My lower back is tense," "My face feels relaxed," or "I feel heat around my core."
7. Once you've finished scanning your entire body, bring your attention to the center of your body around your core or trunk area.

8. Notice what you feel rising from your center. You don't have to try to name anything or search for sensation; just pay attention to any subtle feelings around your core.

9. Notice any thoughts, images, sensations, or emotions that resonate, and just take note of them. Then simply rest.

10. When your timer goes off, open your eyes and stay for another few breaths.

Body scans can help you get to know the full range of physical sensations — some obvious and some not so obvious. In the beginning, you're just getting to know what it feels like to bring your attention to your body. Scans can be done throughout the day. Pause at your desk or in the car, bring your attention to your core section or trunk, and take a few deep breaths. You don't need to put words to what you're experiencing. Just sit with yourself and sense your body. What are you feeling? Is there something you're sensing beneath the array of ordinary physical signals? Over time and with practice, you'll notice deeper sensations beneath the radar of your fast-paced life.

You'll want to start small and keep at it every day. With practice, you'll expand and deepen your fluency. Doing so is how you shift from "kind of feeling" your physical cues to full high-definition sensory experiences. Do a short body scan after you work out, before getting out of bed in the morning, or before turning off the lights in the evening. Listen to the guided Body Scan over and over again.

The more you do it, the better you'll get at discerning how your body informs you. Over time, you'll be able to distinguish between your grumbling hungry stomach and the queasy sense you get there when you're being called to tell the truth in a particular situation, or the excitement you feel at the prospect of eating an ice-cream cone and the surge of energy you get before you sprint your last one hundred meters.

Ask the Question

Trusting the intelligence of your senses takes time and practice. As you keep investigating, you'll strengthen your capacity to decipher your messages. The Body Scan is a great way to develop this capacity. Another effective way to tune in to energy is through inquiry. You learned how to do this in the Verge Practice *Notes to Self.* You ask yourself questions over and over, pausing to listen for any change in energy. The instructions are simple: ask, pause, and listen. You can do this all day long. Here are a few of my favorite questions:

- Can I meet this moment?
- Am I resisting this moment?
- How does my body want to move?
- Am I available?
- Can I be at ease?
- Can I show up?
- Can I let go?

Ask, pause, and listen, and with practice you'll trust in the intelligence emerging from your body. You'll trust its guidance, its alerts and notifications. You'll trust that in every moment your intelligence is reminding you to listen and inviting you to show up and shine.

CHAPTER NINETEEN

Welcoming Peace

In the early 1990s I changed professions from teaching figure skating to teaching and performing on in-line skates, or Rollerblades. I emerged from the cold confines of an ice rink into the world of blacktop and open roads. I was like a cat let out of a cage. I was living in New York City at the time, and Central Park became my palette. I skated every inch of it — hanging on the slalom hill, doing tricks, and dancing with the other performers who made up Team Rollerblade. The sense of freedom was euphoric, but there was something else going on. I experienced a deep sense of peace shining from every cell in my body. When I was on my in-line skates, I felt as if I were coming home.

Peace is closer than you think. It's actually right here waiting to greet you. It's in this moment, and now this one, and now this one. Shift beyond the clutter of your busy mind, and you'll find peace already there waiting. It emerges when you're silent and still. Peace arises not from *doing* more, but from spending more time *being*. Peace emerges in the space between moments, between tasks and conversations, between judging and comparing.

Peace isn't something that happens from getting or achieving; it's a feeling that emerges. It feels eternal. It feels universal and, at the same time, deeply personal. Peace is what you experience when you shift beyond busyness and rest in the space of your natural state. It's the stillness you feel at the end of a long day and the aliveness you feel upon waking the next. Peace is what emerges when you're available for life. It's where you shine — and it may be happening more often than you think.

For me, having peace is the sense of relief I feel when changing into my pajamas and laying my head down on my pillow. It's a cozy feeling I have when both my college-age daughters are home for break. It's feeling rested and refreshed after taking a nap. I also experience peace during challenging situations, such as when I comforted one of my daughters immediately after her first heartbreak or when I sat in silence with my friends as we waited for updates on their missing son, Cayman. I've felt peace in the middle of a thunderstorm, while gazing in awe at the immensity of the night sky, and even when making soup on a cold winter day.

You have more peace in your life than you realize. You may simply need to widen your scope of how you experience it. Know that when you recognize moments of peace, you are living on the verge.

 GUT CHECK:
YOUR EXPERIENCE OF PEACE

Off the top of your head, how do you describe your experiences of being peaceful? What are you doing or who are you with? I gave you some of my examples above. Please write down the first three descriptions that come to mind.

To me being peaceful feels like:

1. _____

2. _____

3. _____

I am peaceful when I am doing this or doing something with this person (or these persons):

1. _____

2. _____

3. _____

Peace-Filled Settings

Most people want to experience more peace and hope they'll find it by achieving something such as a new job, losing ten pounds, or going to a spa. Certain milestones can, of course, bring you temporary peace, but, as you know, once you achieve a milestone, you're off and running to a new one. I've found that peace arises in certain environments, some of which you've already identified in the Gut Check above. Being aware of such environments can help you experience peace more consistently, perhaps more predictably.

Get to know peace, and you'll know what it feels like to shine. The following environments can help you do so:

- Space
- Simplicity
- Stillness
- Silence
- Rhythm

Peace Emerges in Space

Space is a sought-after commodity. We search for space because when we have room to spread out, we feel more settled and at ease — we feel more peaceful. Space can mean sitting in an uncluttered room or driving on a wide-open road. It can mean feeling mentally clear while sky gazing. Space offers us the opportunity to see and think more clearly and shine more brightly. In space, we experience peace.

Imagine you are looking at two possible vacation homes to rent. You walk into the first one to find it so cramped — overstuffed couch and chairs, tables and shelves, heavy curtains, walls covered with pictures, knickknacks everywhere — that you can hardly make your way around. Upon checking out your second prospect, you find it is done in a minimalist Zen design. The walls are white, the furniture sparse, the windows unrestricted, and the few accessories perfectly placed. You immediately feel your shoulders relax, and you start to breathe more deeply. I wonder which one you are going to choose!

Space — whether it's in our physical surroundings, our bodies, or our minds — helps us feel at ease. So creating space in your life can offer you a better chance of experiencing peace more often. You get the idea. More space means more peace. The degree will vary from person to person and situation to situation. Here are a few suggestions for how to create more space in your life.

> Space — whether it's in our physical surroundings, our bodies, or our minds — helps us feel at ease.

Body: You can cultivate space in your body by releasing physical tension through yoga, tai chi, dance, or anything else that gets you moving your limbs. A good sweat is always a great way to cleanse your body and create a feeling of spaciousness throughout.

Mind: As you've learned in various Primer Practices, pausing for a breath or two throughout your day creates space in your mind. It allows you to settle down. Resting, even for a few minutes, is such a great relief that once you do it a few times, you begin looking for opportunities to do it more often in your life. I find ways to pause all the time, especially in transitions such as before getting out of bed, getting out of my car, or diving into my dinner.

Heart: Letting go of your need to force, fix, or flee is an effective way to find emotional space. Drama, whether it's yours or someone else's, crowds your life and drains your energy. Letting go and dropping your drama and need to control open you up and allow the fresh air in.

Physical surroundings: Clear the clutter! Keeping your desk, countertops, and bedroom clean and spacious is a simple and cost-free way to cultivate peace.

Peace Is Found in Simplicity

Peace emerges in the most ordinary moments of life — you may just not be paying close enough attention. Peace is not hard to find when you take the time to show up for your afternoon cup of tea, your bedtime routine, or walking your dog. Peace can be found in the simplicity of an uncomplicated moment. An uncomplicated yoga pose or a slow bike ride can be profoundly peaceful. Give yourself permission to simplify your life, and you'll start noticing opportunities to experience peace in simple moments throughout your day.

You can create more simplicity in your life in the following areas.

Body: Simplify your practices, such as not complicating the Triangle Pose by always having to take a fancy arm variation, allowing a half-hour walk in the evening to be enough of a workout once in a while, or having the courage to sometimes be a beginning student rather than always having to be the expert.

Mind: Mindfulness is a great practice for unraveling the knots in your mind. Pay attention to doing one thing at a time, and you will feel yourself shift beyond your mental noise and have more peace.

Heart: Relationships can get sticky — but they don't have to. By recognizing that drama drains you, you can look for ways to simplify your relationships. Being honest is a great way to keep your life simple.

Physical surroundings: Simplifying your surroundings is like creating space. Less stuff and more beauty in your surroundings create an optimal environment for having more peace. Look at your physical surroundings at home, work, and even in your car. Keep only what is essential and let go of the rest.

Peace Arises from Stillness

Stillness is a key ingredient in experiencing more peace in your life. There's no way around it. Taking the time to be still in your daily life is one of the greatest gifts you can give yourself.

Body: The five-minute resting pose at the end of a yoga class is a great example of how accessible stillness is in your life. Physical stillness is often the best place to start. Step out of the rat race and give yourself permission to stop moving. You'll start breathing more deeply almost immediately. You may not realize that you never stop moving until you do.

> Taking the time to be still in your daily life is one of the greatest gifts you can give yourself.

Mind: Your busy mind likes to stay, well, busy. When you're racing through life, you're not necessarily looking for ways to slow down, until you do. Your Verge Practices are all helpful ways to become familiar with stillness and how to find more of it in your life.

Heart: Emotional stillness can feel like the sweet relief of taking a long hot shower or a long walk in the woods. Not trying to control can help you settle emotional disturbance more quickly. This doesn't mean you're going to be emotionless; in fact, it means looking at your emotions directly, acknowledging them — anger, disappointment, and sadness — and allowing them to pass.

Physical surroundings: Ah, this is my favorite. There's no better place to experience physical stillness than in nature. Even though the wind may blow and the ocean roar, there's still a deep stillness that settles your nerve endings. Lie down in the grass or on the beach, float in a pool, or sit on a park bench, and you'll feel the sense of peace arise from deep within you.

Peace Can Be Felt in Silence

I feel the same way about silence that I do about stillness. There's no doubt that silence is incredibly overlooked in our culture. Silence cultivates peace. It settles you in a way that opens you up wide to glimpsing peace in every pocket of your life.

Silence cultivates peace.

We're bombarded with noise everywhere we turn. Since this is not going away, you're going to need to make finding silence a priority in your life. Give yourself five minutes in silence, and you'll feel a sense of peace rise up to greet you — just five minutes. Here's how.

Body: Physical silence is much like stillness. Take the time to pause, allow your body to settle. Silence in your body is also found by taking time to be alone. Find opportunities to exercise, walk, or eat alone in silence. You'll feel your body unwind from even an hour in silence. As you do, your body becomes an instrument, a channel for experiencing peace.

Mind: There's really nothing like silence to settle your mind. Being quiet is hugely undervalued in our society. Remember the Italian expression *Che dolce far niente*, which translates as "How sweet it is to do nothing." This is what silence feels like, sweet and empty. I've spent days in silence and can honestly say I've never experienced such peace as when I allow myself to be quiet.

Heart: Similar to stillness, emotional silence arises when you allow everything to be as it is. When you give other people freedom to be as they are, you will, in turn, have the freedom to be as you are. This is peace. Let go and allow, over and over, and you will tap into the silence of your heart, where your sense of peace flourishes like nowhere else.

Physical surroundings: Finding silence in your physical surroundings is not only easy; it's a must. There is noise, noise everywhere, and nobody is going to offer you silence; you've got to find it yourself. Set reminders to turn down the noisemakers — radio, television, and computers — during the day, and you'll find peace waiting in the silence.

Peace Emerges in Rhythm

Gentle, slow rhythm opens you to experience peace in your life. Breath, movement, stillness, and silence are powerful ways to synchronize your mind and body and cultivate peace. Take a look.

Body: Being in sync cultivates peace. Moving in rhythm, such as walking, dancing, skating, skiing, and swimming, creates a sense of harmony and alignment in your systems. Synchronize your mind and body through breath and movement and use rhythm to have more peace.

Mind: As you synchronize your mind and body by focusing on your breath and watching your thoughts, you'll slow down the rhythm of your brain waves from beta to alpha. The slower the brain waves, the greater the overall sense of peace you experience.

Heart: Your heartbeat is always thumping. Sometimes it's irregular, and sometimes it's slow and rhythmic. New studies have been looking at heart-rate variability, or HRV — the beat-to-beat changes in your heart rate. When your HRV is smooth and balanced, in other words, not irregular, you are in a synchronized state. This evokes a deep sense of well-being. Synchronizing your mind and body through breath, movement, stillness, and silence can establish a smooth HRV.

Physical surroundings: The rhythm of nature is life's most brilliant symphony. Pause to listen to the rhythm of the ocean or the song of the crickets or the bullfrogs, and within minutes you'll feel peace emerge.

Peace emerges when you shift beyond your busy mind. It arises from space, simplicity, stillness, silence, and rhythm. It feels like coming home.

Peace can be found in every moment and in every breath. Recognize peace in the predictable environments, and you'll then start to see them appear in the not-so-obvious moments. I've found peace in the most unpredictable situations, like flying down the streets of New York City on my Rollerblades.

CHAPTER TWENTY

Experiencing Fearlessness

From Rollerblading and hip-hop aerobics to yoga, I was that high-energy kick-ass teacher you had to have energy to train with. I got you fired up to push your limits, face your fears, and transform your life. That was before opening my yoga center twelve years ago, when I signed a lease and hired a bunch of new teachers. I went from a kick-ass freelancer to a director and a boss. I focused on attendance and quality control. I even tempered my teaching style so I wouldn't stand out among my team. I wanted everyone to shine, but I had a few things yet to learn about being a leader and about fearlessness.

Fearlessness is like a clean-burning fire, shedding light upon — and blazing through — every role, responsibility, and relationship that is not congruent. Be fearless, and you'll uncover everything false or imbalanced in your life. You expose what isn't real and true. You lean into the uncomfortable and unfamiliar. You embrace. You let go. You show up and shine.

Be fearless and face your perceived fears head-on — all of them — including your phobias, anxiety, trepidation, nervousness, worry, and restlessness. Sense them in your body before they take hold of your life. Be willing to see, touch, smell, and taste every morsel of fear. Stare at what you think you fear

Stare at what you think you fear most, and it will weaken.

most, and it will weaken. Meet it with confidence, and you nip it in the bud before it sabotages the moment.

Fearlessness pervades every move you make and every word you speak. When you're fearless, you're neither too hard nor too soft. You're anything but weak and a far cry from overpowering. Being fearless has a quality of transparency when you speak from the heart. You are truthful in a way that uncovers what's not fair. You are genuine in your appreciation for life and sincere in how you move about the world.

One glimpse of fearlessness, and you'll know it. It feels crisp and clear, like opening the window on a winter day. Being fearless lifts you up and invigorates you. It has momentum. Do it once, and you know you can do it again — you'll want to be fearless again and again. Being fearless makes you feel awake and fully alive. Being fearless definitely makes you show up and shine.

Pay attention and recognize opportunities to be fearless emerging in your life today. They will come in many packages; they will sometimes be subtle and sometimes bold. Here are some examples to wet your whistle. Choose those you'd like more of in your life and add them to the reminders in your *Notes to Self* practice. Fearlessness is:

Telling the truth even when your voice shakes
Being genuine
Acknowledging others
Going above and beyond
Dropping drama
Being silent and still
Being available
Leaning into the unknown and unfamiliar
Being humble
Pressing into the edge of your comfort zone

Listening deeply without giving advice

Admitting you're wrong

Taking responsibility

Asking for help

Bringing Fearlessness into Your Practice

You can bring fearlessness into your practices and become familiar with what it feels like to really look at yourself under a microscope. The best practices to do this, to stare at thoughts, emotions, and the habits of your mind, are your mindfulness practices. This includes your toolbox of Primer Practices in *Notice This Moment* and your seated meditation practice, *Meet My Mind*.

Use your practices to learn how your busy mind works and how it has been dictating your behavior. Examine what arises and passes with keen interest. Leave no stone unturned. Look directly at your busy mind until you burn through it or see through it to the space beyond it. Rest in the space of your unconditioned clear mind until thoughts emerge again, until busyness returns, and then burn through it again. Do this over and over again. Small glimpses, many times. Be honest, kind, and sincere in your efforts, and your glimpses will extend into longer experiences.

Get to know how your busy mind works, and you'll understand how life works. Become familiar with your tendencies, and you'll compassionately recognize them in others. Practice patience and kindness toward yourself, and in turn you will become patient and kind toward others. This is how your heart opens. When you touch the center of your own heart, you open yourself to be touched by the world.

Fearlessness is neither too hard nor too soft, and it reveals in you the beautiful qualities of genuineness and truthfulness. You live more in the "we" and less in the "me."

Truthfulness

To understand truthfulness it's helpful to first see what is not true. Being truthful is your willingness to investigate — *everything*. Everything you think, say, and do in private and in public is food for growth. It all counts. Notice your beliefs and behaviors. Face everything. Avoid nothing. Open all your closet doors, and don't leave any stone unturned. Being fearless is to walk through life shining the torch of truthfulness in every corner. It's all up for investigation, every last negative thought about how you look, the whispers under your breath, even the seemingly small shortcut you took at work. It all counts.

Face everything.
Avoid nothing.

You can try to be honest with yourself in your everyday busy life, but it's challenging to get to the root of what's true or untrue in the middle of the chaos. In order to really look, you need to shift your perspective. You can't be truthful from your busy mind, because you can't see clearly from your busy mind. Finding space, stillness, and silence is the most direct way to tease apart the knots that bind you and block you. Get quiet and settle into the space where you will see clearly, and you'll get an honest look at how you operate.

Be willing to recognize behaviors and beliefs that shut you down and hold you back. Uncover those things and times that feel sticky. Be willing to sense what feels untrue and unkind. Why not expose it all? The only things you have to lose are the habits that weigh you down and clutter up your busy mind.

Investigate insecurity enough, and it weakens and eventually dissolves. Face anxiety enough, and you'll sense it coming before it takes hold of your day. Get to know what you believe, how you're conditioned, how you judge, what your behaviors look like. Investigate everything. This fearless way of living, this truthfulness, opens you up to experiencing life like never before.

Truthfulness feels clean — that's how you instinctively recognize it. It feels precise, whole, complete. It feels fresh. In the unconditioned space of your clear mind you move and speak with intention. Your actions and words are sincere. You carry a quality of excellence with you into all that you do and in all that you are. Carry the torch of truthfulness into the world, and you meet life head-on with openness and availability. This is fearlessness, and it's exactly how you show up and shine.

Genuineness

A special quality of being emerges from truthful living. You begin to appreciate the joy of being awake and fully alive. Look directly at your tendencies to gossip, worry, or control, and eventually you'll get really tired of living like that. Get to know your busy mind, and you'll eventually see right through your patterns of selfishness and manipulation.

No longer satisfied with hiding or sneaking around, you seek out opportunities to be honest and open. You fall in love with living in the clean space where you're naturally and effortlessly clear, bright, and open, and you refuse to go back. No longer willing to carry the burdens of your busy mind, you lay down your ammunition and drop your masks. You rest in the space of pure awareness, where you're neither too hard nor too soft. You embrace each moment as an opportunity to shine.

Genuineness is how being fearless emerges when you're willing to touch those hard-to-get-to places deep down inside. In touching these spots that may be filled with hurt, rejection, and betrayal, you begin to soften and open to the world. Despite everything that's happening in your life — the problems and relationships, the ups and downs — when you are genuine, you meet life and those in it with appreciation and cheerfulness.

To me, being genuine feels like wrapping a soft blanket

around myself and then opening my heart to the world. I have nothing to protect and everything to give. I experience life beyond drama, where there's nothing to gain and nothing to lose. In this space I feel joyful and free. I am open and available to meet life head-on, to show up fully, and to shine brightly.

In touching these spots that may be filled with hurt, rejection, and betrayal, you begin to soften and open to the world.

Truthfulness and genuineness emerge in the space beyond your busy mind. Study your busy mind and get to know how it operates. Be willing to expose it all and to experience the truth. Be willing to investigate your beliefs and behaviors, and you'll experience what lies beyond them. You'll slip into the unconditioned space where you move with intention and speak with compassion.

To be fearless is to face your perceived fears, to sense them in your body, and to meet them with confidence. In so doing, you discover how to shift past them into the space where you're already genuine and truthful, into the space where you're already awake and fully alive.

Before becoming a leader, I thought I knew what it meant to be fearless. Now I recognize that the kick-ass teacher filled with "spit and vinegar" has evolved. Now I show up and shine in a whole new way. I've learned to face everything and avoid nothing. I've opened my heart to the world and now move with a fearlessness that's more genuine and more truthful, that is not too hard and not too soft, that is more "we" and less "me."

Conclusion

There's a gap, a split second of time when you're not quite in the past and not quite in the future. Right here, this exact moment, you have a choice. You can remain asleep or wake up. You can stay locked in your busy mind, consumed by stuff to do and places to be, or you can show up. In every moment, the decision is yours to make: speed right by this moment, or choose to be here right now. The verge — this exact moment — is waiting for you. All you need to do is wake up and show up — and you will shine in your life like never before.

You don't need me to tell you how and you don't need this book to show you the way. You already know how to be awake — you glimpse life in high definition all the time. You already know how to be fully alive — you experience high-voltage energy all the time.

On the Verge is a call to be awake and fully alive. It was not written to be a one-and-done book, and it's not just a summary of tools and techniques for you to try a few times and toss. My intention is not to assign you more things to do or to pack your schedule with more activities. I hope to spark your curiosity and empower you to investigate the clarity, vitality, and confidence that naturally and effortlessly emerge in the unconditioned space just beyond your mental clutter and emotional baggage. I hope to get you fired up about directly experiencing your life by being awake and fully alive not just once in a while, but every day, on purpose.

The Verge Practices I offer are a road map to get to know your busy mind and to shift beyond it, where you glimpse your naturally clear mind, bright body, and open heart. The Verge Strategies I offer are a set of inquiries to help you stay awake and aware — to live on the verge consistently.

So practice, practice, practice. Remember, small glimpses, many times. Don't take on too much too fast. Ease in slowly. It's really important to start small, stay steady, and build from there. Be kind and patient. Bookmark the At-a-Glance practice pages, so you can go back and reread them, especially as you get started. Set practice reminders on your phone. Don't forget to check out the Verge Mobile App and seek live teachers for continued support.

As your practices grow and as your strategies become your way of living, you'll live on the verge more frequently, trusting that your direct experiences are real, that you already have what you need to be awake and fully alive, and that you already know how to show up and shine.

But no one can do this for you. No one can show up for you. Only you can. Only you can directly experience your life. Only you can live on the verge, and the great news is you can start doing so right now.

Pause for a moment. Take a few deep breaths, and take in your surroundings. Look around, listen, smell, hear, and touch it all, as if for the first time. Notice your body and the intelligence flowing through you. Look at your busy mind. Now look right through your mind and see what lies beyond the drama and distraction. Look straight through the veil of thoughts and emotions and notice the space beyond it. Give yourself permission to rest in this space — the place where you're already clear, bright, and open, where you're already awake and fully alive. Smile. You have arrived. In this space, you are on a threshold. In this exact moment — between a moment ago and a moment from now — you are on the verge.

Acknowledgments

I trust that, along the way, we touch each other with our spark of aliveness. Every encounter and experience counts. So many people have crossed my path, each one in some way guiding me to arrive at this place. If you are one of them, I thank you for encouraging me to show up and shine.

To my rock-star team of women: You redefine what it means to be excellent. I would like to thank Lisa Tener, for her fearless guidance with my proposal; Rita Rosenkranz, my agent, who never let me settle for ordinary; Kelly Malone, whose delightful editing style kept me smiling when I wanted to cry; and Georgia Hughes, my editor at New World Library, whose encouraging words and gentle kindness helped me to lean in when I wanted to run away.

To my teachers: Although *On the Verge* is primarily about my experiences, I would have never been able to make any sense of them without your help. I thank my incredible meditation teachers, Scott and Nancy McBride of ClearLight Meditation, and mentors Michael Carroll, Lori Hanau, Fran Sorin, and Bonnita Roy; my first yoga teachers, Beryl Bender Birch, Thom Birch, and Baron Baptiste; and those teachers who transformed my life but whom I've never met, Adyashanti, Pema Chödrön, Eckhart Tolle, and Caroline Myss.

To my kindred spirits and fellow yogi travelers who share my enthusiasm for practice, specifically Jane Rosato, Kristin Page, Michelle Baldino, Erica Bleznak, Johnny Gillespie, Jennifer Schelter, Ann Martin, Michelle Kosvitch, Dan Thompson, Rolf Gates, Kelly McNelis Senegor, and all the teachers of Verge Yoga past and current: Each of you has stretched me and cracked me open in some way, helping me to face everything and continue to grow.

To coaches Andy Talley, of Villanova football; Jay Wright, of Villanova basketball; Pat Chambers, of Penn State Basketball; and Danielle Fagan: Thank you for trusting me with your student athletes.

To my students along the way, especially to those at Verge Yoga: Thank you for allowing me to explore and experiment with insights for this book.

To my four parents, Charles and Eleanor Ferrara and Sam and Lucy Bradley; and my two brothers, Tom and Bob: thank you for demonstrating what it means to love and be kind and for giving me a remarkably strong and stable foundation from which to fly.

To my husband, Brian, for reading and rereading my manuscript and for patiently listening to me go on and on during our long evening walks. You are my greatest cheerleader and my most honest critic. I'm blessed to be experiencing life by your side.

And finally to my beautiful daughters, Christina and Julianna, my greatest gifts, who inspire my life and make me feel awake and fully alive every day. Being along for your journey has opened me to mine.

Online Practice Support

Establishing new practices can be challenging, which is why it's necessary to have support. The Verge Mobile App will support you with guided audio, video practices, reminders, and other fun stuff. Download the app through www.carabradley.net.

Here's what you'll find on the Verge Mobile App. Some are included on the free app and some on the premium app you can buy for a nominal fee.

Audio

Primer Practices

Stop, Take Five, Experience
Wake-Up Call
Sky Gazing
Distracted or Right Here Right Now?
Remember the View
Box Breathing
Counting Breath
Coming Home
Body Scan

Meet My Mind

Meditation Instruction
Focused Deep Breathing 10-Minute Practice
Focused Deep Breathing 20-Minute Practice

Be Kind

Making Friends with Yourself (guided meditation)

Video

Move My Body

Mindful Movement (guided all-levels movement practice)
Beginner Yoga (guided beginner yoga practice)
Synchronizing Mind and Body (guided all-levels yoga practice)

Timers and Reminders

Move My Body Practice Timer
Meet My Mind Practice Timer
Notes to Self Reminders, Intentions, and Questions

About the Author

Cara Bradley, a former pro skater for Team Rollerblade, is a lifelong teacher, mental strength coach, and entrepreneur who has devoted more than three decades to movement disciplines and personal transformation. As the founder of Verge Yoga in suburban Philadelphia, she spends her time coaching thousands of students, including CEOs and professional athletes, to settle down, show up, and realize their potential. Dubbed the "secret weapon" for the Villanova University football team's 2009 FCS National Championship, Cara trains athletes to have "fierce focus" and composure in the fires of competition.

Cara is the host of the podcast *Real Women, Courageous Wisdom* for Women For One, a series featuring Truthtellers — everyday women passionate about sharing their journeys and inspiring others. She shares her personal journey and discoveries in her popular weekly blog, *Cara Bradley Unveiled*.

Cara presents talks and yoga and mindfulness programs at conferences and universities nationwide and offers on-demand classes and international retreats. She cofounded the nonprofit Mindfulness Through Movement, which provides full-year mindfulness programs to schools in Philadelphia. She is a Certified Strength and Conditioning Specialist (CSCS) for the National Strength and Conditioning Association and a Yoga Alliance

Experienced Registered Yoga Teacher (E-RYT). She lives in Wayne, Pennsylvania, with her husband, her dog, and, on occasion, her two world-traveling daughters. Connect with Cara by emailing fullyalive@carabradley.net or through one of the following sites.

www.carabradley.net
www.vergeyogacenter.com

 Facebook: **carabradleyteacher**

 Twitter: **carabradley16**

 LinkedIn: **carabradley**

 Google+: **carabradley**

 Instagram: **carabradleyunveiled**

 YouTube: **Cara Bradley**

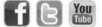